Simulation and Surgical Competency

Guest Editors

NEAL E. SEYMOUR, MD
DANIEL J. SCOTT, MD

SURGICAL CLINICS OF NORTH AMERICA

www.surgical.theclinics.com

Consulting Editor
RONALD F. MARTIN, MD

June 2010 • Volume 90 • Number 3

SAUNDERS an imprint of ELSEVIER, Inc.

W.B. SAUNDERS COMPANY

A Division of Elsevier Inc.

1600 John F. Kennedy Blvd., Suite 1800, Philadelphia, PA 19103-2899

http://www.theclinics.com

SURGICAL CLINICS OF NORTH AMERICA Volume 90, Number 3

June 2010 ISSN 0039–6109, ISBN-13: 978-1-4377-1877-5

Editor: Catherine Bewick

Surgical Clinics of North America (ISSN 0039–6109) is published bimonthly by Elsevier Inc., 360 Park Avenue South, New York, NY 10010-1710. Months of publication are February, April, June, August, October, and December. Business and Editorial Offices: 1600 John F. Kennedy Blvd., Suite 1800, Philadelphia, PA 19103-2899. Periodicals postage paid at New York, NY and additional mailing offices. Subscription prices are $291.00 per year for US individuals, $475.00 per year for US institutions, $145.00 per year for US students and residents, $356.00 per year for Canadian individuals, $590.00 per year for Canadian institutions, $401.00 for international individuals, $590.00 per year for international institutions and $200.00 per year for Canadian and foreign students/residents. To receive student/resident rate, orders must be accompanied by name of affiliated institution, date of term, and the *signature* of program/residency coordinator on institution letterhead. Orders will be billed at individual rate until proof of status is received. Foreign air speed delivery is included in all *Clinics* subscription prices. All prices are subject to change without notice. POSTMASTER: Send address changes to *Surgical Clinics*, Elsevier Health Sciences Division, Subscription Customer Service, 3251 Riverport Lane, Maryland Heights, MO 63043. **Customer Service (orders, claims, online, change of address): Telephone: 1-800-654-2452 (U.S. and Canada); 314-447-8871 (outside U.S. and Canada). Fax: 314-447-8029. E-mail: journalscustomerservice-usa@elsevier.com (for print support); journalsonlinesupport-usa@elsevier.com (for online support).**

Reprints. For copies of 100 or more, of articles in this publication, please contact the Commercial Reprints Department, Elsevier Inc., 360 Park Avenue South, New York, New York 10010-1710. Tel. (212) 633-3812, Fax: (212) 462-1935, e-mail: reprints@elsevier.com.

The Surgical Clinics of North America is also published in Spanish by McGraw-Hill Interamericana Editores S.A., P.O. Box 5-237 06500 Mexico D.F. Mexico; and in Portuguese by Interlivros Edicoes Ltda., Rua Comandante Coelho 1085, CEP 21250, Rio de Janeiro, Brazil; and in Greek by Paschalidis Medical Publications, Athens Greece.

The Surgical Clinics of North America is covered in *MEDLINE/PubMed (Index Medicus), EMBASE/Excerpta Medica, Current Contents/Clinical Medicine, Current Contents/Life Sciences, Science Citation Index,* and *ISI/BIOMED.*

Printed and bound by CPI Group (UK) Ltd, Croydon, CR0 4YY

Transferred to Digital Print 2012

Contributors

CONSULTING EDITOR

RONALD F. MARTIN, MD
Staff Surgeon, Department of Surgery, Marshfield Clinic, Marshfield, Wisconsin;
Clinical Associate Professor, University of Wisconsin School of Medicine and Public
Health, Madison, Wisconsin; Colonel, Medical Corps, United States Army Reserve

GUEST EDITORS

NEAL E. SEYMOUR, MD
Professor, Tufts University School of Medicine; Chief, Division of General Surgery,
Vice Chair Department of Surgery, Baystate Medical Center; Director, Baystate Simulation
Center-Goldberg Surgical Skills Laboratory, Springfield, Massachusetts

DANIEL J. SCOTT, MD
Associate Professor, Frank H. Kidd Jr, MD Distinguished Professorship in Surgery;
Director, Southwestern Center for Minimally Invasive Surgery UT, Southwestern Medical
Center, Dallas, Texas

AUTHORS

RAJESH AGGARWAL, PhD, MA, MRCS
Division of Surgery, Department of Surgery and Cancer, Imperial College London,
St Mary's Hospital, London, United Kingdom

CLINT BOWERS, PhD
Professor, Department of Psychology, University of Central Florida, Orlando, Florida

L. MICHAEL BRUNT, MD
Professor, Department of Surgery, Washington University School of Medicine, Saint Louis,
Missouri

JO BUYSKE, MD
Associate Executive Director, American Board of Surgery; Adjunct Professor of Surgery,
University of Pennsylvania School of Medicine, Philadelphia, Pennsylvania

JANIS A. CANNON-BOWERS, PhD
Research Professor, Institute for Simulation and Training, University of Central Florida,
Orlando, Florida

IAN CHOY, MD
Department of Surgery, University of Toronto, Toronto, Ontario, Canada

BRIAN J. DUNKIN, MD
Professor of Clinical Surgery, Department of Surgery, The Methodist Hospital, Weill Cornell Medical College, Houston, Texas

GARY DUNNINGTON, MD, FACS
J. Roland Folse Professor and Chair, Department of Surgery, Southern Illinois University School of Medicine, Springfield, Illinois

GERALD M. FRIED, MD
Chairman, Professor of Surgery, Adair Family Chair of Surgical Education, Department of Surgery, McGill University Health Centre, McGill University, Montreal, Quebec, Canada

TEODOR P. GRANTCHAROV, MD, PhD
Assistant Professor, Department of Surgery, St Michael's Hospital, University of Toronto, Toronto, Ontario, Canada

MARY E. KLINGENSMITH, MD
Professor, Department of Surgery, Washington University School of Medicine, Saint Louis, Missouri

JEFFREY M. MARKS, MD
Director of Surgical Endoscopy, Associate Professor, Department of Surgery, University Hospitals, Case Medical Center, Cleveland, Ohio

ANDREAS H. MEIER, MD
Associate Professor of Surgery and Pediatrics, Medical Director, Surgical Skills Center; Chairman, Division of Pediatric Surgery, Department of Surgery, Southern Illinois University, Springfield, Illinois

ALLAN OKRAINEC, MD, MHPE
Department of Surgery, University of Toronto; Division of General Surgery, Toronto Western Hospital-University Health Network, Toronto, Ontario, Canada

JOHN T. PAIGE, MD
Assistant Professor of Clinical Surgery, Department of Surgery, Louisiana State University School of Medicine, New Orleans, Louisiana

VANESSA N. PALTER, MD
Research Fellow, The Wilson Centre, Toronto General Hospital, Toronto, Ontario, Canada

KATELYN PROCCI, BS
Doctoral Student, Department of Psychology, University of Central Florida, Orlando, Florida

HILARY SANFEY, MB, BCh, FACS
Professor of Surgery and Vice Chair for Educational Affairs, Department of Surgery, Southern Illinois University School of Medicine, Springfield, Illinois

RICHARD M. SATAVA, MD, FACS
Professor, Department of Surgery, University of Washington Medical Center, Seattle, Washington; Senior Science Advisor, US Army Medical Research and Material Command, Fort Detrick, Maryland

DIMITRIOS STEFANIDIS, MD, PhD, FACS
Clinical Assistant Professor of Surgery, University of North Carolina; Medical Director, Carolinas Simulation Center, Division of Gastrointestinal and Minimally Invasive Surgery Department of General Surgery, Carolinas Medical Center, Charlotte, North Carolina

COLIN SUGDEN, MRCS
Clinical Research Fellow, Division of Surgery, Department of Surgery and Cancer, Imperial College London, St Mary's Hospital, London, United Kingdom

MELINA C. VASSILIOU, MD, MEd
Assistant Professor of Surgery, Department of Surgery, McGill University Health Centre, McGill University, Montreal, Quebec, Canada

Contents

The apprenticeship model that surgical training has traditionally relied on has proven to be an expensive, time-consuming, and inconsistent model for producing skilled surgeons. Combined with increased public scrutiny on patient safety, financial concerns, restricted work hours, and expanding skill requirements, it has become clear that a new pedagogic paradigm is required. This article reviews the evidence supporting the need and justification of simulation in surgical education and explores the existing and potential roles of simulation in the training and evaluation of future surgeons.

Increasingly, trainees are being exposed to simulators for the purpose of acquiring surgical skills. This article addresses the theoretical framework behind surgical skill acquisition and explores the factors that optimize learning on simulators. Furthermore, this article evaluates the role of currently used performance metrics for documentation of skills proficiency and provides suggestions for the incorporation of additional, more sensitive performance metrics that may lead to improved transfer of simulator-acquired skill.

In the last 2 decades, surgical education has experienced a transformative paradigm shift from the purely service-based Halstedian system to a curriculum-driven model based on educational theory. With the advent of minimally invasive surgery and its educational challenges, fostered by the simultaneously occurring rapid advances of computer technology and graphics and further promoted by rising concerns about patient safety, simulation and skills training has become a well-established tool in the arsenal of the surgical educator. Although most training institutions now have access to skills laboratories and simulation centers, running and integrating these facilities into the surgical curriculum remains a challenge. This article outlines general principles that are relevant for training facilities of all sizes and covers aspects from the initial phase of planning and

Several factors, including reduced resident work hours and concerns for patient safety, have led to the introduction of dedicated skills laboratories and a more widespread belief in the value of time spent in skills training. The American College of Surgeons and the Association of Program Directors in Surgery established a three-phase skills curriculum for all surgery residents. Phase 1 involves basic surgical skills instructional modules and a Verification of Proficiency assessment. After undergoing teaching and practice sessions in the authors' skills lab, all first-year surgical residents (post graduate year 1 residents) from general surgery and four surgical specialty programs are tested on 11 non-specialty specific basic surgical skills before performing these in clinical situations.

This article focuses on key aspects of the "nontraditional" surgical subjects of organizational structure and team interaction. First, the deficiencies in team dynamics found within the modern operating room (OR) and their resultant consequences are highlighted. Next, essential human factors concepts related to error generation, organizational culture, high reliability, and team science as applied to the OR environment are reviewed. Finally, various strategies for improving OR team function, including the use of high-fidelity simulation (HFS) in team training are discussed.

Simulation-based training is rapidly becoming an integral part of surgical training. However, the effectiveness of this type of training is as dependent on the manner in which it is implemented and delivered as it is on the simulator itself. In this article, the authors identify specific elements from the science of learning and human performance that may assist educators in optimizing the effects of simulation-based training. These elements include scenario design, feedback, conditions of practice, and others. Specific guidelines for simulation-based surgical training are provided.

With recent concerns regarding patient safety, and legislation regarding resident work hours, it is accepted that a certain amount of surgical skills training will transition to the surgical skills laboratory. Virtual reality offers enormous potential to enhance technical and non-technical skills training outside the operating room. Virtual-reality systems range from basic low-fidelity devices to highly complex virtual environments. These systems can act as training and assessment tools, with the learned skills effectively transferring to an analogous clinical situation. Recent developments

THE CLINICS ARE NOW AVAILABLE ONLINE!

Access your subscription at:
www.theclinics.com

Foreword

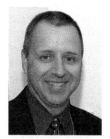

Ronald F. Martin, MD
Consulting Editor

Legend has it that Charlie Chaplin once entered a contest for the best impersonation of Charlie Chaplin and took third place. I can only assume that the two more highly regarded participants were quite good or that, perhaps, the judges knew less about Charlie Chaplin than might have been ideal.

Before I render further comment I should make a few disclaimers. As some readers may be aware, I serve as a reservist in the United States Army. We in the Army believe in simulation to the point where we have giant parcels of land on which we participate in exceptionally high-fidelity simulation on a large and very expensive scale. I also serve on occasion as an examiner for the American Board of Surgery (ABS) where I participate in a simulation of sorts for the certifying examination. I also serve as a program director in surgery where I require and participate in the simulation training of residents and faculty. So I state unequivocally up front that I espouse a belief that surgical simulation is of value in training surgeons. But one never puts forth disclaimers unless one is about to rock the boat a bit—so here goes.

Simulators most likely will have an increasing role in the training of surgeons for a variety of reasons. During this period of transition, however, there are a few things that must be put on the table for discussion. For instance, I have been to meetings where it has been stated that a surgeon cannot achieve competence without the use of simulators in training. Perhaps the speaker was trying to make a strong point, but this statement, simply put, is not true. Many generations of surgeons have been trained without formal simulation training, other than on a previous patient and perhaps cadavers or in animal laboratories (maybe those can be counted as support of the speaker's comment), and the majority of the advancement of our craft came from these surgeons. So, surgeons can be trained without simulators.

Those comments notwithstanding, it is highly likely that surgical simulation will ease transitions for learners and teachers in the acquisition and transfer of skill sets. A low-stakes environment with high fidelity produces an optimal setting to learn potentially

Surg Clin N Am 90 (2010) xiii–xv
doi:10.1016/j.suc.2010.04.002
0039-6109/10/$ – see front matter © 2010 Elsevier Inc. All rights reserved.

dangerous procedures, and the compressed time frame of simulation may be a huge benefit in the training of residents in the current era of work hour restrictions.

The addition of access to simulator environments requirements to training programs in surgery brings another area of concern—Should the use of simulators be considered part of the 80-hour workweek for residents? On one hand, the use of simulators may be a time saver in training but on the other hand it does add another task to fit into a crowded workweek. As the requirements for simulation increase, the demands on resident time and faculty time are likely to become more difficult to integrate into the overall work flow, not to mention the financial impact.

Outside the purview of resident surgeon training, the use of simulators for assessing competence or maintenance of certification (MOC) may be even thornier. The ABS, in its original charter, states that its function is "to protect the public and improve the specialty." As Dr Buyske writes in this issue, "The ABS Booklet of Information, published annually, further notes that the specific objective of the ABS is 'to pass judgment on the education, training, and knowledge of broadly qualified and responsible surgeons'." And by passing judgment, the ABS adds another metric for people to use as a proxy measure for surgeon competency (refer to earlier disclaimers—on the whole I believe this a good thing). This presents an interesting dilemma, however: Is testing the best way to measure and assess competency?

I stated previously that I believe that simulation is of value in training surgeons and that I believe in the overall process of training and assessing surgeon performance and board certification—and I stand by it. But if beliefs were good enough to base high-stakes decisions on, there would be no need for science. It has been argued in this and in previous issues of the *Surgical Clinics of North America* that MOC will improve patient safety. It has also been argued that the use of simulators will improve patient safety. But to the best of my knowledge a tool or process has not been constructed to assess whether or not those concepts are true. The addition of MOC and mandatory use of simulators adds a monetary cost and a time cost to trainees and practicing surgeons alike. At some point, if the principles of evidence-based surgery are adhered to, the impact of these changes will have to be assessed, and whether or not improvement in care divided by these additional costs is deemed worthwhile (a sort of impact value equation) will have to be determined. Furthermore, the value of ABS MOC, with or without simulation, may have to be compared to the real-time tracking of surgeon performance via quality control/quality improvement programs, such as the National Surgical Quality Improvement Program or institutional or third-party payer data to see which is a better marker of competency or quality.

Simulators are here. Simulators are going to have an increased role in the lives of surgeons for the foreseeable future. The role of simulation is likely to expand beyond the organ-surgeon or patient-surgeon interface and enter the realm of team and institutional simulation in a meaningful way in the near future. There is a great deal to be learned from colleagues in the aviation and transportation industries about simulation. It is a lot easier, however, to build a simulator for a Boeing 737 after having designed and built the original Boeing 737 than it is to build a human simulator. And one lesson that must be learned from colleagues in the military about simulation is that no battle plan, no matter how carefully planned and trained, survives first contact with the enemy.

This issue, edited by Drs Seymour and Scott, contains some spectacular material from some of the most respected leaders not only in surgical simulation but also in our surgical discipline. I am deeply appreciative of their efforts in developing this volume. Whether the reader is a medical student, a resident or fellow in training, a practicing surgeon, or responsible for training and large systems, this issue brings invaluable material. Perhaps in a decade or two we can look back and see how all this turns out. Let us hope that we currently know more about simulation than the aforementioned judges knew about Charlie Chaplin.

Ronald F. Martin, MD
Department of Surgery
Marshfield Clinic
1000 North Oak Avenue
Marshfield, WI 54449, USA

E-mail address:
martin.ronald@marshfieldclinic.org

Preface

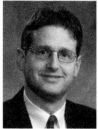 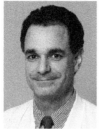

Neal E. Seymour, MD   Daniel J. Scott, MD
Guest Editors

The concept of surgical competency represents an exceedingly complex construct that may defy clear definition. Efforts have been made in the course of postgraduate residency education, however, to define competency areas that collectively speak to this complex construct. By reframing training in terms of patient care, medical knowledge, practice-based learning and improvement, interpersonal and communication skills, professionalism, and systems-based practice competencies, the Accreditation Council for Graduate Medical Education has categorized areas that must be addressed with specific educational interventions, which remain largely undefined. Among all the possible interventions, medical simulation has emerged from the realm of technical curiosity to become a mainstream and now mandatory component of training. Its role in helping to achieve and clearly demonstrate surgical competency is an evolving one. There is no prescriptive roadmap to have surgeons render simulated clinical care, in the form of technical task performance or complex decision making, in order to address competency concerns. The number of programs using simulation training methods and the number of surgeons who have been exposed to some form of simulation, however, continue to grow. Even in the absence of broad directives, the stage has been set for an array of simulation training methods to occur outside of residency, and active speculation has been prompted as to how this might eventually shape future certification processes.

We, the editors of this edition of *Surgical Clinics of North America*, feel that surgical stimulation offers an opportunity for educators to effectively impart skill and to facilitate the certification of competency. This view may be somewhat controversial. The current technologic status of surgical stimulation imposes important limitations on what can be simulated as well as to whom the simulated experiences can be delivered. It is not unreasonable to expect that this situation will change, particularly if the demand for simulation at all levels of fidelity increases in the near future. There is evidence that changes on the user demand side are already occurring. Our aims in assembling the contents of this edition are to give the *Surgical Clinics of North America* readership a comprehensive view of the state-of-the-art of simulation use in surgery and a vision

Surg Clin N Am 90 (2010) xvii–xviii
doi:10.1016/j.suc.2010.04.001   **surgical.theclinics.com**

of how ongoing and future developments in connection with ever-expanding use may influence achievement and certification of surgical competency.

Neal E. Seymour, MD
Division of General Surgery
Department of Surgery
Baystate Medical Center
759 Chestnut Street, Springfield, MA 01199, USA

Daniel J. Scott, MD
Southwestern Center for Minimally Invasive Surgery UT
Southwestern Medical Center
5323 Harry Hines Boulevard
Dallas, TX 75390-9156, USA

E-mail addresses:
neal.seymour@baystatehealth.org (N.E. Seymour)
Daniel.Scott@UTSouthwestern.edu (D.J. Scott)

Simulation in Surgery: Perfecting the Practice

Ian Choy, MD[a], Allan Okrainec, MD, MHPE[a,b],*

KEYWORDS

- Simulation • Surgical training • Surgical education
- Surgical skills

A NEED FOR SIMULATION

All improvements are illusory and temporary if knowledge, experience, and skills cannot be or are not transmitted to future generations of practitioners of the art and science of surgery.

—*Ambroise Paré 1510–1590.*

Practical Considerations

William Halstead's model of surgical education has faithfully and effectively trained countless generations of surgeons, successfully sustaining the art and science of surgery. Halstead's apprenticeship-based residency program has endured essentially unaltered from that which he started at Johns Hopkins University in 1889. This is particularly impressive, considering the rate and extent of change that the medical profession has undergone during this same period. Recently, however, cracks in the foundations of our pedagogical system have become increasingly difficult to ignore, with a growing body of literature calling for the need for change.[1,2] Although the traditional residency model appears to have been able to keep up with the advances in skills, technology, and science thus far, the recent constellation of pressures on this system including increased public scrutiny, financial concerns, restricted work hours, and expanded skill requirements threatens to produce residents who may, for the first time, be less skilled than the previous generation.[2]

The seminal work of Kohn and colleagues[3] drew attention to the issue of preventable medical errors. Quoting a rate of 44,000 to 98,000 deaths per year in the United

Financial disclosures: None.

[a] Department of Surgery, The Banting Institute, University of Toronto, 100 College Street, Room 311, Toronto, ON M5G 1L5, Canada

[b] Division of General Surgery, Toronto Western Hospital-University Health Network, 8MP-325, 399 Bathurst Street, Toronto, ON M5T 2S8, Canada

* Corresponding author. Division of General Surgery, Toronto Western Hospital-University Health Network, 8MP-325, 399 Bathurst Street, Toronto, ON M5T 2S8, Canada.

E-mail address: allan.okrainec@uhn.on.ca

Surg Clin N Am 90 (2010) 457–473

doi:10.1016/j.suc.2010.02.011

0039-6109/10/$ – see front matter © 2010 Elsevier Inc. All rights reserved.

surgical.theclinics.com

States associated with medical errors, the investigators brought this issue well beyond the medical community to society at large.[4] To put these figures into perspective, 44,000 deaths per year exceed the number of fatalities from motor-vehicle accidents, breast cancer, or AIDS. Increased public emphasis on patient safety and reducing medical errors has raised ethical concerns about trainees learning basic skills on patients. This issue has led to calls for a separation of practice from performance.[5,6]

The increasing costs associated with health care have also become a major concern. In 1999, it was estimated that the additional cost to train a surgical resident in the operating room (OR) for 4 years was nearly $50,000.[7] Adding to these costs are the increased complication rates seen with junior residents compared with their senior colleagues as shown in multiple studies.[8,9]

Restricted work hours have also had a significant impact on surgical residency programs; the practice remains a contentious issue. The recent European Working Time Directive, implemented in August 2009, has further reduced the number of hours that a resident can work, from 56 to 48 hours a week, including overtime and a minimum uninterrupted 24-hour rest period per week and 11 hours per day.[2,10] Similarly, the Residency Review Committee (RRC) in the United States introduced the 80-hour workweek in 2003[11] to all accredited medical training institutions. States such as New York have had comparable regulations in place as early as 1989, after the Libby Zion case.[12] Whereas the reduction of work hours affects residents from all specialties, surgical residents are particularly vulnerable to such changes given the technical nature of the field.

With the development of new technology and surgical techniques, residents have been required to develop more skills in less time. Minimally invasive and endoluminal therapies have forced residents to acquire a unique set of psychomotor skills adding further pressure to an already stressed curriculum. Furthermore, as residents dedicated a greater proportion of their time to these new procedures, their experience and knowledge of more traditional open procedures has decreased. Schulman and colleagues[13] in 2007 reviewed the case logs of surgical residents and found that out of the 745 laparoscopic cholecystectomies that were performed at their institution, only 39 required conversion to an open procedure. The researchers concluded that the low number of conversions and open bile duct explorations for gallstones inadequately prepared residents in these procedures. Livingston and Rege[14] also demonstrated in 2005 that with the introduction of endoscopic retrograde cholangio-pancreatography and a subsequent decrease in the number of common bile duct explorations (CDEs), there was a marked increase in the complication rate associated with CDEs. The investigators suggested that new treatment algorithms should be instituted to take into account these high complication rates and that residency programs should incorporate dedicated training modules into surgical residencies.

Changes in what we teach, and how we teach, are clearly needed to counteract these challenges. Patient safety requires a more robust and accountable system. Restricted work hours and increasing costs mean that efficiency must be a priority. Changes in technology and skills requirements will necessitate novel pedagogical techniques. Fortunately, such reforms have already been introduced. Psychomotor skills training has been introduced in Canada and the United States as early as the 1960s, whereas in England similar workshops were introduced in the mid-1970s.[15] In 1998, the University of Toronto opened the Surgical Skills Centre at Mount Sinai Hospital. The rationale for the creation of the center was to provide an environment wherein trainees could accrue technical skills in a pedagogically sound setting. The initial mission of the center was to change the way fundamental surgical skills were taught and evaluated, to provide a platform for continuing education in surgical skills, and to create a laboratory for research and development of surgical skills innovation. The center inaugurated a formalized curriculum for skills training for surgery residents and developed validated feedback and performance assessment ratings.[6,15–19] The success of these programs, combined with the rapid adoption of laparoscopy and increasing concerns regarding credentialing, has contributed to the growing recognition of the importance of simulation as a training tool.

Challenges of the Laparoscope

Aside from the practical considerations for the need of simulation in surgical education, the advent of laparoscopic surgery has presented some unique technical and sociologic challenges that did not exist in traditional open surgery. Depth perception is significantly affected because of the transformation of a 3-dimensional surgical space into a 2-dimensional video image. Trainees must learn to adapt to this new interface by learning how to use cues in the 2-dimensional image to determine spatial relationships between structures. The fulcrum effect, caused by fixed trocar sites for instrument access, represents another psychomotor challenge for trainees, as it requires the surgeon's hand to move in a direction opposite to that of the instrument. Laparoscopy also uses long instruments that separate the surgeon's hand from the anatomic structures, significantly reducing tactile feedback. As such, trainees must develop new cues from these laparoscopic instruments to determine when they are grasping too hard or pulling too vigorously. Finally, as there is less direct interaction between both of the surgeon's hands, trainees have a tendency to ignore their nondominant hand. This reduces efficiency and can lead to potentially dangerous surgical technique.

There are also sociologic challenges that have been introduced into the OR environment with the advent of minimally invasive surgery (MIS), which have been addressed at a more theoretical level. Charles Perrow, a sociologist at Yale University, has applied his teamwork theoretical concepts to the field of surgery.[20] He studied the differences between the types of social interaction in laparoscopic and open surgery and described 2 characteristics of teamwork systems: coupling and interactive complexity. Coupling describes the degree to which the various actors in a system rely on each other. A tightly coupled system contains actors whose roles depend a great deal on each other and who require a strong central authority to efficiently direct resources. Surgery is a tightly coupled system: scrub nurses, surgical assistants, and anesthesiologists work closely together with the surgeon in an environment where seconds can mean the difference between life and death. Although the tasks of each actor may be simple, a tightly coupled system dictates that each individual is essential to the overall success of the operation.

Interactive complexity describes the level of interaction between actors. A low level of complexity indicates that actors in a system are able to perform their tasks independently from each other, requiring minimal communication. Alternatively, a highly complex system involves constant communication and coordination between multiple actors. Highly complex systems require a decentralized authority, allowing the actor's direct involvement in processes, as well as the ability to collectively respond to unexpected problems.

Open surgery is tightly coupled but low in interactive complexity; both systems require a strong centralized authority. This system is ideal for resident training, as residents do not require much skill to participate in an operation, and instruction and control is unidirectional. Laparoscopic surgery differs from open surgery in that it is both tightly coupled and highly complex. This leads to competing and contradictory demands on leadership. With the introduction of video laparoscopy, surgical assistants became more important to the success of the procedure, as they assumed more active roles. Information flow ceased being unidirectional, as surgeons became increasingly dependent on the information provided by assistants. The implication of these changes to medical students and residents was that to actively participate in laparoscopic procedures, trainees needed to arrive in the OR already equipped with a basic set of laparoscopic skills. These skills would therefore have to be acquired via pretraining.

Pretraining is extremely beneficial because of the unique technical requirements of laparoscopic surgery. Gallagher and colleagues[21] describe a conceptual framework on learning modules for MIS training that is based on the concept of an individual's finite capacity for attention.[22] Gallagher gives the example of a novice surgeon who has not undergone any prior skills training. In the OR, residents are faced with an overwhelming array of tasks. Some of these skills can be acquired independently of the OR, such as psychomotor performance, depth perception, and spatial judgment. The more-cognitive skills are OR dependent, such as operative judgment, comprehending instructions, and gaining additional knowledge associated with the OR environment. As **Fig. 1** illustrates, the combination of these tasks may easily meet or exceed the trainee's attentional capacity threshold.

By pretraining novices on tasks that are not OR dependent, trainees are able to automate these skills. When these previously trained novices participate in the OR, they are able to dedicate less of their attentional resources to these automated tasks and can then focus more of their attention toward OR-dependent tasks.

Whether it be restricted working hours for residents, socioeconomic pressures, complexity of laparoscopic procedures, or maximizing the learning potential of surgical trainees, it is clear that changes must be made in the way that future surgeons are educated. Although no single solution holds the key to solving these educational dilemmas, simulators will almost certainly play a significant role. The various characteristics of simulators that make them uniquely suited to dealing with improving

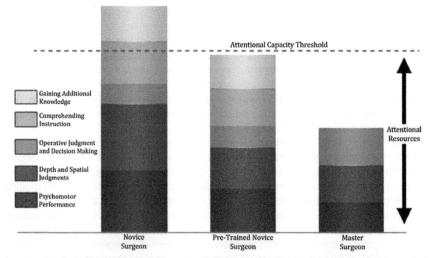

Fig. 1. Hypothetical attentional resource benefits of simulation training. *Modified from* Gallagher AG, Ritter EM, Champion H, et al. Virtual reality simulation for the operating room: proficiency-based training as a paradigm shift in surgical skills training. Ann Surg 2005;241(2):367; with permission.

residency training and addressing the aforementioned issues are reviewed in the following sections.

DEVELOPING A CURRICULUM

Skills training and simulation in surgical education have evolved dramatically over the past 2 decades and have gained widespread acceptance as a valuable educational tool. However, before curriculum development could take place, the important task of evaluating surgical skills had to first be laid out.

Traditionally, skill assessment was performed directly by the attending surgeon through the use of In-Training Evaluation Reports (ITERs), and learning curves were reported as a function of the number of procedures performed. However, ITERs are rife with central tendency errors, the "halo effect," and recall bias.[23] Furthermore, as most surgeons can attest, basing competence on the number of procedures performed is, at best, a crude indicator of actual performance. As skills training gained more attention, it became obvious that a new assessment method was needed. Before any determination can be made regarding the effectiveness of a training tool, a trainee's skill level had to be quantified, thus providing an evidence-based support for new curricula.[24,25]

The Global Assessment Scale has received the most attention in the area of skills assessment and has been shown through numerous studies to be an effective tool in that regard. One of the most widely cited global assessment scales is the Objective Structured Assessment of Technical Skills (OSATS) developed at the University of Toronto.[16] It is based on a 5-point grading scale of 7 performance metrics including respect for tissue, time and motion, instrument handling, knowledge of instruments, use of assistants, flow of operation, and knowledge of the specific procedure. Ultimately this tool was found to have a moderate-to-high interrater reliability and demonstrated construct validity for live and bench models.[16] The use of the OSATS tool has expanded beyond general surgery, and the tool is used throughout the various surgical specialties. OSATS has also proven to be a useful tool in simulation research to help determine the effectiveness of various educational interventions and the transferability of skills learned.

OSATS, however, was not developed or validated for the assessment of laparoscopic skills. With the growing influence of laparoscopic surgery and the lack of evidence demonstrating the transferability of skills from laparoscopic simulators, Vassiliou and colleagues[23] at McGill University, in 2005, built on the OSATS model and developed a rating scale called the Global Operative Assessment of Laparoscopic Skills. Initially described for assessment of skills during laparoscopic cholecystectomy, this tool has also been validated for use in other laparoscopic procedures.[26]

With increasing evidence supporting the use of simulation in surgical skills training, the RRC mandated that by the end of 2008, every surgical residency program in the United States must have a skills curriculum. However, as late as 2006, Korndorffer and colleagues[27] showed that although 85% of residency programs considered skills training laboratories effective in improving OR performance, only 55% of the 162 programs surveyed actually had a skills laboratory. Moreover, only 89 (55%) of these 162 programs actually had mandatory training requirements. Clearly, the work of curriculum change continues to be ongoing.

In an attempt to provide more guidance in this area, the American College of Surgeons (ACS) and the Association of Program Directors in Surgery (APDS), led by Drs Dunnington, MacRae, and DaRosa, developed the Surgical Skills Curriculum in 2005.[11] Based on the American College of Graduate Medical Education core competencies, this curriculum was designed to meet RRC requirements while also being affordable and portable. The basic model of this curriculum is to have multiple modules structured around video tutorials, followed by guided practice until a performance goal has been achieved; assessment is then made using global rating scales. These modules are divided into 3 phases. Phase I, based on basic core skills and tasks, was released in 2007. Phases II and III, focusing on advanced skills and team-based skills, respectively, were released in 2008.

The Surgical Skills Curriculum has gone a long way in addressing the need for a standardized simulation-based program. The curriculum is available free of cost via the Internet, and it has the potential to significantly improve on the number of skills laboratories available to residents as well as the number of residents who use them.

SIMULATORS
Animal/Cadaver Models

The earliest simulations used for laparoscopic surgery were animal and cadaver models. Although initially used for the development of laparoscopic instruments and techniques, animal models were well suited for training. Before other simulators were developed, animal and cadaver models were the only methods available for hands-on training. However, legal and ethical issues and the cost and labor-intensive nature of these models have restricted the frequency of their use. Thus, their use was often limited to short, single-practice sessions contrary to the distributed learning model shown to improve skill retention.[28] Furthermore, animal and cadaver models were also limited in their ability to model pathology, and variations in their normal anatomy made them difficult to be used as an objective performance assessment and in their subsequent use in monitoring of trainee progress over time.

To provide further evidence of the decreased need for the use of animal models, in 1997, Martin and colleagues compared surgical skills training on live animal models with that on bench models using the OSATS assessment score. Comparing the performance of 5 tasks including excision of a skin lesion, hand-sewn bowel anastomosis, stapled bowel anastomosis, T-tube insertion, control of *inferior vena cava* hemorrhage, and abdominal wall closure, Martin showed that the ability of both methods to measure surgical skills were equivalent.[16] Animal and cadaver models, however, continue to be used today under specific circumstances such as the development of novel procedures and techniques, including natural orifice transluminal endoscopic surgery (NOTES).[29,30]

Video Trainers

Video (box) trainers (VT) were developed soon after the proliferation of laparoscopic surgery as the need arose for better skills training. Although VTs lack the anatomic accuracy of animal models, they provided an inexpensive, efficient, and reproducible environment for basic laparoscopic skills training. VTs ranged in complexity from cardboard boxes to elaborate all-in-one devices, but they all share the same simple design of a video camera, a monitor, and a box with access points for instruments. Various groups and manufacturers developed their own systems and skill modules, but 3 in particular were the most widely adopted.

In 1992, James Rosser introduced the Top Gun Laparoscopic Skills and Suturing Course, also known as the Yale Laparoscopic Skills and Suturing Program. The program focuses on providing an effective and entertaining approach to acquiring the necessary instrument dexterity for laparoscopic suturing. The course consists of 3 drills. The *rope pass* requires the participant to pass a rope between 2 grasping instruments by manipulating alternating 1-in colored areas. The *cup drop* requires the participant to use alternating hands to drop peas into a cup through a small hole from a distance of approximately 1 cm. The *triangle transfer drill* requires the participant to transfer a wooden triangle back and forth across a field using 2 needle drivers loaded with a curved needle.[31] Once participants have practiced these 3 drills, they can then more effectively practice laparoscopic suturing with intracorporeal knot tying using a similar VT model setup.

Scott and colleagues[32] subsequently expanded on the Yale tasks, creating the guided endoscopic modules, also known as the Southwestern stations (**Fig. 2**).

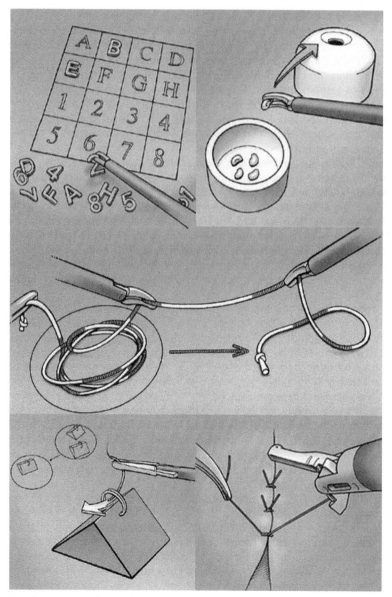

Fig. 2. Southwestern station tasks.

The 3 aforementioned Yale tasks were modified such that an assistant was not needed; in addition, a checkerboard drill was added, which involves placing 16 block letters and numbers in their appropriate marked locations on a map, as well as a foam suturing task. One of the landmark studies in the development of VTs came in 2000, when Scott and colleagues[32] first demonstrated transferability of skills from a VT to the OR environment. In this study, 23 postgraduate year 2 and 3 surgery residents were randomized to receive basic skills training on the Southwestern stations for 30 minutes daily for 10 days or no simulator training at all. All residents underwent pretest and posttest assessment on the VT and in the OR during a laparoscopic cholecystectomy.

Scored using the OSATS tool, the researchers found that although there was no difference in pretest scores, the posttest scores showed a significant improvement in the laboratory and in the OR. They found that VT-trained residents had improved scores on 4 of the 8 OSATS criteria including respect for tissue, instrument handling, use of assistants, and overall performance. Three of the 8 criteria, time and motion, knowledge of instruments, and flow of operation, although not reaching statistical significance, did show a strong trend toward improvement. The only criteria that showed no difference was knowledge of operation, a result that one might expect with a training program that does not contain a cognitive component.

In 1998, Fried and colleagues[5,33–35] from McGill University developed the McGill Inanimate System for Training and Evaluation of Laparoscopic Skills (MISTELS) program. To develop this simulator, a panel of experienced laparoscopic surgeons were gathered, who, after reviewing video records of several laparoscopic cholecystectomies, appendectomies, inguinal hernia repairs, and Nissen fundoplications, identified 7 specific skill domains that would be the most appropriate for training and evaluation. These skills include magnified monocular vision and limited depth perception, visual-spatial perception, use of both hands in a complementary manner, securing of a tubular structure using a ligating loop, precise cutting while using the nondominant hand for counter-traction, suturing using extracorporeal knots, and suturing using intracorporeal knots.

These domains were then refined into a set of 5 tasks: peg transfer, pattern cutting, placement and securing a ligating loop around a foam appendage, simple suturing and extracorporeal knot tying, and simple suturing and intracorporeal knot tying (**Fig. 3**). Evaluation of these tasks was performed using a combination of time and accuracy. After the development of MISTELS, there has been an extensive body of research confirming the construct, face, predictive, and transfer validity of this simulator as a training and assessment tool.[5,34,36–40] The supporting evidence of the efficacy of VTs as a training tool has led to widespread adoption of these simulators by organizations such as the ACS/APDS and the RRC, as discussed earlier. Furthermore, the success of the MISTELS program in particular garnered the attention of the Society of American Gastrointestinal and Endoscopic Surgeons (SAGES) in 1998. At that time, SAGES was developing their own laparoscopic training course and chose to incorporate MISTELS with their own cognitive curriculum. The Fundamentals of Laparoscopic Surgery (FLS) program is the product of this collaboration.[41] It consists of a cognitive component presented in 5 Web-based modules (preoperative considerations, intraoperative considerations, basic laparoscopic procedures, postoperative considerations, and manual skills instruction and practice), a simulation-based technical skills component adapted from the 5 MISTELS tasks, and an assessment component that measures both cognitive and technical skills.[42] FLS itself has also achieved widespread acceptance. In 2008, the American Board of Surgery (ABS) announced that applicants would also be required to obtain FLS certification before

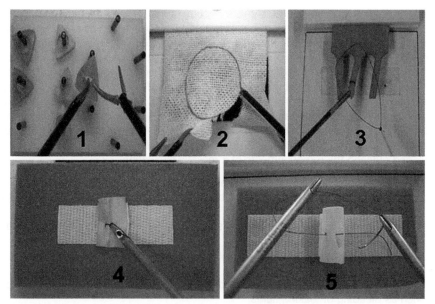

Fig. 3. Fundamentals of laparoscopic surgery tasks. (1) Peg transfer. (2) Pattern cutting. (3) Placement and securing of ligating loop. (4) Simple suturing and extracorporeal knot tying. (5) Intracorporeal knot tying.

taking the ABS examination.[43,44] FLS training programs have been set up across North America, and they have also become very popular throughout the developing world, opening up huge possibilities in the realm of international laparoscopic skills development.[45]

Virtual Reality Simulators

Virtual reality (VR) simulators have undergone significant advances during the past decade and now provide several significant advantages over animal models and VTs. As a computer-based technology, VR simulators are able to model full surgical procedures, with anatomic accuracy and diversity. Although some physical simulators have incorporated full procedures such as colectomies,[46] these models are often expensive and are not reusable. VR simulators can have a high initial cost, but there are few recurring costs for repeated use other than maintenance, and adding additional procedural simulations involves simply installing another program on the existing hardware. VR simulators also have the benefit of automation, whereby training instructions and feedback can be programmed into the simulation. Again, automated metric devices have been developed for physical simulators, such as the Imperial College Surgical Assessment Device (ICSAD)[47,48]; however, VR simulators are able to provide a greater variety of measurements. By using automated metrics, trainees may obtain instantaneous and frequent performance assessments without the constant presence of a trained surgeon.

VR simulation has been in use for several decades in other fields, rooted in the large-scale development of simulators for the aviation industry in the 1940s to help meet the training requirements and demands for pilots in World War II.[49] Training using VR simulators is essential for pilots, as it allows them to practice critical maneuvers under widely variable and often extremely rare circumstances. These simulators are also extremely useful for more routine maneuvers, as they allow for easy repetition and practice without the high costs and safety risks associated with flying actual aircraft. Outside of the medical industry, the benefits of VR simulation have long been acknowledged and have been adapted for other industries as the technology has advanced. For instance, one finds VR simulators in varied fields, from aerospace and military applications to mining equipment and urban planning. Even within other areas of the medical profession, VR has been used in treating patients with various phobias.

Only within the last decade have surgeons leveraged the capabilities of VR as a training tool. Richard Satava first proposed the use of VR in surgical education in 1993 and outlined the 5 requirements of a realistic simulation.[50]

1. Fidelity—the image must have sufficiently high resolution to appear real.
2. Object properties—the organs must deform when grasped and must fall with gravity.
3. Interactivity—the surgeon's hand and surgical instruments must interact realistically with the organs.
4. Sensory input—force feedback, tactility, and pressure must be felt by the surgeons.
5. Reactivity—the organs must have appropriate reactions to manipulation or cutting, such as bleeding or leaking fluids.

Along with the advantages inherent in VT simulators (repetition, cost-effectiveness), VR simulators are also able to simulate entire anatomic environments under a range of conditions and levels of difficulty. With this improved fidelity over VTs, VR simulators are better able to meet Satava's requirements. Furthermore, the ability to provide detailed isometric feedback on measures such as time, number of instrument movements, and path length makes VR simulators capable assessment tools. The need for the expensive and time-consuming role of an expert evaluator is therefore potentially eliminated.

Since the late 1990s, multiple VR simulators have become available in the market. Like the VTs, 3 VR simulators in particular have been the focus of most research in this area.[51] One of the earliest of these VR simulators is the MIST-VR (Mentice, Gothenburg, Sweden). Recent models have incorporated force feedback or haptics into this system, but earlier models consisted of 2 nonhaptic instrument handles, a computer, and a monitor. Being one of the earliest VR simulators on the market, MIST-VR has also become one of the most established, with a number of studies demonstrating the construct validity, reliability, and transferability of the system.[52–56] Seymour and colleagues[52] in 2002 published the first landmark study demonstrating transferability of skills from the VR to the OR after training on the MIST-VR system. Using 16 surgical residents in a randomized double-blind study, results showed that VR-trained residents were 29% faster and 6 times less likely to commit an error at performing a gallbladder dissection, whereas non–VR-trained colleagues were 9 times more likely to transiently fail to make progress.[52] At present, the MIST-VR system is used to focus solely on tasks, and a procedural component has not yet been developed.

LapSim (Surgical Sciences, Göteborg, Sweden) is similar in design to the MIST-VR, with 2 instrument handles, a computer, and a monitor. LapSim was also initially used to focus on tasks such as coordination, cutting, clipping, dissection, and suturing, and tasks similar to the FLS program have recently been incorporated. The use of LapSim also provides an anatomic environment, allowing procedural simulations such as laparoscopic cholecystectomies and a variety of gynecologic procedures such as salpingectomy, tubotomy, and tubal occlusion to be performed.

LAPMentor (Simbionix, Cleveland, OH, USA) has hardware components slightly different than that of the LapSim and MIST-VR systems. Along with 2 haptic instrument handles, a computer, and a screen, there is also a camera control incorporated into the design. Similar to the LapSim system, the software component contains both basic skills modules as well as various procedure modules, including laparoscopic cholecystectomy, ventral hernia repair, sigmoid colectomy, and gastric bypass (**Fig. 4**). The procedure modules also contain multiple variations to simulate aberrant anatomy and disease states.

Graphics, haptics, tasks, procedure modules, and metrics have all undergone significant change and improvement since the first VR simulators were developed. These changes are important to take into account when reviewing the literature, as they can have important effects on a trainee's experience. As an example, studies have shown that for VR simulators without haptics, residents actually prefer the VT for tasks such as suturing.[57] However, subsequent studies have demonstrated improved face validity, speed, and accuracy with haptics than without.[58] Although several review articles have been published attempting to summarize the literature on the efficacy of VR simulators, those results and conclusions are likely to change over time because of the evolving nature of the technology.[50,59]

As an assessment tool, multiple studies have demonstrated the construct validity of VR simulators using a combination of time, global assessment score, and device metrics.[60–62] McDougall and colleagues[62] in 2006 demonstrated using the LAPMentor system that the device metrics were able to discriminate between novice and skilled surgeons. However, results also showed that not all simulated tasks were equal in this regard. More difficult tasks possessed increased discrimination. At the same time, the validity of some of these device-generated isometric data has been brought into question. In 2008, Andretta and colleagues[63] evaluated the metrics used by the LAPMentor system and found that they were not able to discriminate between levels of expertise. That said, motion analysis devices such as the ICSAD, as well as VT and VR simulators, have been used in both open and laparoscopic environments and have been shown to be a valid measure of dexterity, correlating well with global rating scales.[47,48,55]

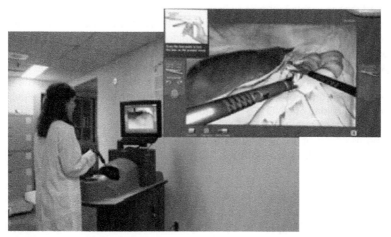

Fig. 4. Simbionix LAPMentor system, with a trainee performing a full procedure laparoscopic gastric bypass simulation (*inset*).

VR simulators have demonstrated a clear benefit over no training, with studies showing a significant improvement in time, accuracy, number of errors, and overall score.[52,64–66] Similarly, as an adjunct to standard laparoscopic training, VR simulation has been shown to decrease operating time, significantly decrease errors, improve composite scores, and improve economy of movement.[51] When compared with VTs, the benefits of VR are less clear. In terms of training basic skills on VR simulators without haptics, most studies show either equivalence or just a slight improvement with VR.[51,54,55,59] Again, the applicability of these studies to today's VR simulators can be questioned and likely requires further study.

Overall, results seem to support the use of VR simulators. As technology matures and becomes more cost-effective, incorporating VR simulators into residency curricula may become more practical. However, as Gurusamy and colleagues[51] noted, incorporating simulators into surgery curricula may necessitate a decrease in the amount of time that residents dedicate to standard training, a cost-benefit tradeoff which has yet to be addressed in any of the literature, and is likely be a growing focus as the supporting evidence for simulation increases.

EVOLVING FIELDS
Team Simulation

Team simulation, sometimes referred to as high-fidelity simulation, involves the immersion of participants into an entire simulated environment, which allows for the process of learning to occur in context.[67,68] In surgery, this has been achieved by recreating entire OR suites, complete with nursing and anesthetic staff. Team simulation incorporates the teaching of surgical skills with OR team skills, such as communication, vigilance, decision-making, and effective leadership.[69] With many of the advantages inherent in surgical simulators (training in a learner-friendly environment, ability to mimic low-frequency, high-risk events), team simulation is likely to be another important tool in future surgical curricula.

Natural Orifice Transluminal Endoscopic Surgery

NOTES is a recently emerging experimental alternative to open and laparoscopic surgery. Through the use of transluminal incisions, abdominal wounds are avoided. Recent advances in this technology have expanded the possibilities of this technique beyond transsigmoid appendectomies and transgastric cholecystectomies[70] to include transvaginal gastric lymphatic mapping[29] and Roux-en-Y gastric bypass.[71] Although several technical challenges still exist, such as reliable methods to close the insertion site and optimization of the instrument interface,[72] one of the main challenges to the widespread adoption of NOTES is the development of adequate training facilities.[73] Gillen and colleagues,[73] in 2009, have already developed and established the construct validity of a NOTES simulator called the endoscopic-laparoscopic interdisciplinary training entity, modeled after the VTs described previously. However, given the flexibility of VR simulators and NOTES, it is only a matter of time before computerized models are developed.

Telesimulation

Telementoring, teleproctoring, and telesimulation all describe aspects of teaching and assessing skills remotely through the use of cameras, video monitors, and microphones. Similar technology is already widely used in health care through telemedicine, allowing physicians and surgeons to treat and follow up with patients who live in more remote or underserviced areas. Telementoring specifically involves a mentee performing a surgical procedure under the guidance of a mentor who, while being able to provide real-time feedback, is in a different physical location and in unable to actually physically intervene. Several groups have already demonstrated the feasibility and effectiveness of telementoring in surgery.[74–76]

Telesimulation is different from telementoring in that the mentee performs simulated tasks rather than operate on a real patient. This requires that both the instructor and the trainee have simulators that are connected over the Internet using videoconferencing software. With a series of other computers and webcams, the instructor and trainee are able to see themselves as well as their respective simulations in real time. This setup allows the learner to observe the correct manner in which a specific skill is to be performed by the remote instructor, followed by repetitive practice of that particular skill by the trainee while the instructor observes and corrects errors in real time (**Fig. 5**). This training platform was developed by the authors' group at the University of Toronto in response to a need for more regular and distributed training of laparoscopic skills in resource-poor countries.[45,77] A recent study comparing telesimulation with self-practice in a group of surgeons in Botswana has shown that telesimulation is a very effective method of teaching laparoscopic skills using the FLS simulator, with 100% of participants in the telesimulation group achieving a skills certification pass rate compared with only 38% in the self-practice group.[77] Since then, the telesimulation program has expanded and is now being used to teach surgical as well as other medical skills in various countries around the world.

In the future, these methods of distance learning will become increasingly relevant, with the ongoing adoption of laparoscopic procedures in remote communities, development of new minimally invasive equipment such as NOTES, ongoing globalization of health care, and increased social awareness of disadvantaged communities both globally and nationally.

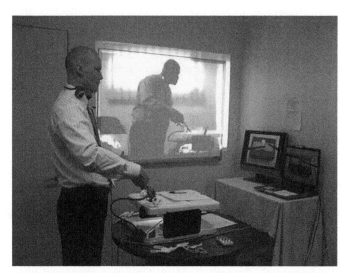

Fig. 5. A surgeon in Toronto teaches laparoscopic suturing to a surgeon in Botswana using telesimulation. *Modified from* Okrainec A, Smith L, Azzie G. Surgical simulation in Africa: the feasibility and impact of a 3-day fundamentals of laparoscopic surgery course. Surg Endosc 2009;24(2):418; with permission.

SUMMARY

The increasing pace of scientific and technologic innovation has opened an array of opportunities to heal through surgical intervention. Transferring this expanding set of skills and knowledge to future generations in the setting of increased public scrutiny, limited financial resources, restricted work hours, and limited exposure to rare procedures presents a formidable challenge. Simulation training and competency-based curricula offer an opportunity to improve current training models to address these challenges and create effective, efficient, and safe residency programs.

REFERENCES

1. Reznick RK, MacRae H. Teaching surgical skills–changes in the wind [see comment]. N Engl J Med 2006;355(25):2664–9.
2. Grantcharov TP, Reznick RK. Training tomorrow's surgeons: what are we looking for and how can we achieve it? ANZ J Surg 2009;79:104–7.
3. Kohn KT, Corrigan JM, Donaldson MS. To err is human: building a safer heath system. Washington, DC: National Academy Press; 1999.
4. Leape LL, Berwick DM. Five years after to err is human: what have we learned? [see comment]. JAMA 2005;293(19):2384–90.
5. Fried GM, Feldman LS, Vassiliou MC, et al. Proving the value of simulation in laparoscopic surgery. Ann Surg 2004;240:518–28.
6. Tsuda S, Scott D. Surgical skills training and simulation. Curr Probl Surg 2009;46: 271–370.
7. Bridges M, Diamond DL. The financial impact of teaching surgical residents in the operating room. Am J Surg 1999;177:28–32.
8. Wilkiemeyer M, Pappas TN, Giobbie-Hurder A, et al. Does resident post graduate year influence the outcomes of inguinal hernia repair? Ann Surg 2005;241: 879–84.
9. Kauvar DS, Braswell A, Brown BD, et al. Influence of resident and attending surgeon seniority on operative performance in laparoscopic cholecystectomy. J Surg Res 2006;132(2):159–63.
10. What is the European working time directive? Available at: http://www.dh.gov.uk/en/Managingyourorganisation/Humanresourcesandtraining/Modernisingworkforceplanninghome/Europeanworkingtimedirective/DH_077304. Accessed September 15, 2009.
11. Scott DJ, Dunnington GL. The new ACS/APDS skills curriculum: moving the learning curve out of the operating room. J Gastrointest Surg 2008;12:213–21.
12. Strongwater AM. Transition to the eighty-hour resident work schedule. J Bone Joint Surg Am 2003;85:1170–2.
13. Schulman CI, Levi J, Sleeman D, et al. Are we training our residents to perform open gall bladder and common bile duct operations? J Surg Res 2007;142(2): 246–9.
14. Livingston EH, Rege RV. Technical complications are rising as common duct exploration is becoming rare. J Am Coll Surg 2005;201(3):426–33.
15. Anastakis DJ, Wanzel KR, Brown MH, et al. Evaluating the effectiveness of a 2-year curriculum in a surgical skills center. Am J Surg 2002;185:378–85.
16. Martin JA, Regehr G, Reznick R, et al. Objective structured assessment of technical skills (OSATS) for surgical residents. Br J Surg 1997;84:273–8.
17. Reznick R, Regehr G, MacRae H, et al. Testing technical skill via an innovative "Bench Station" examination. Am J Surg 1996;172:226–30.

18. Lossing A, Hatswell E, Gilas T, et al. A technical-skills course for 1st-year residents in general surgery: a descriptive study. Can J Surg 1992;35(5):536–40.
19. Matsumoto ED, Hamstra SJ, Radomski SB, et al. A novel approach to endourological training: training at the surgical skills center. J Urol 2001;166:1261–6.
20. Zetka JR. Surgeons and the scope. Ithaca (NY): Cornell University Press; 2003.
21. Gallagher AG, Ritter EM, Champion H, et al. Virtual reality simulation for the operating room: proficiency-based training as a paradigm shift in surgical skills training. Ann Surg 2005;241(2):364–72.
22. Broadbent D. Selective and control processes. Cognition 1981;10:53–8.
23. Vassiliou MC, Feldman LS, Andrew CG, et al. A global assessment tool for evaluation of intraoperative laparoscopic skills. Am J Surg 2005;190:107–13.
24. Darzi A, Smith S, Taffinder N. Assessing operative skill. BMJ 1999;318:887–8.
25. Shah J, Darzi A. Surgical skills assessment: an ongoing debate. BJU Int 2001;88: 655–60.
26. Gumbs AA, Hogle NJ, Fowler DL. Evaluation of resident laparoscopic performance using global operative assessment of laparoscopic skills. J Am Coll Surg 2007;204(2):308–13.
27. Korndorffer JR, Stefanidis D, Scott DJ. Laparoscopic skills laboratories: current assessment and a call for resident training standards. Am J Surg 2006;191: 17–22.
28. Moulton C-A, Dubrowski A, MacRae H, et al. Teaching technical skills: what kind of practice makes perfect? a randomized controlled trial. Ann Surg 2006;244: 400–9.
29. Cahill RA, Asakuma M, Perretta S, et al. Gastric lymphatic mapping for sentinel node biopsy by natural orifice transluminal endoscopic surgery. Surg Endosc 2009;23(5):1110–6.
30. Asakuma M, Perretta S, Allemann P, et al. Challenges and lessons learned from NOTES cholecystectomy initial experience: a stepwise approach from the laboratory to clinical application. J Hepatobiliary Pancreat Surg 2009;16(3):249–54.
31. Rosser JC, Davis BR, Qureshi HN. Intracorporeal suturing: the top gun experience. In: Fischer JE, Bland KI, editors, Mastery of surgery, vol. 2. Philadelphia (PA): Lippincott Williams & Wilkins; 2007. p. 2592.
32. Scott DJ, Bergen PC, Rege RV, et al. Laparoscopic training on bench models: better and more cost effective than operating room experience? J Am Coll Surg 2000;191(3):272–83.
33. Derossis AM, Fried GM, Abrahamowicz M, et al. Development of a model for training and evaluation of laparoscopic skills. Am J Surg 1998;175(6):482–7.
34. Derossis AM, Bothwell J, Sigman HH, et al. The effect of practice on performance in a laparoscopic simulator. Surg Endosc 1998;12(9):1117–20.
35. Fraser SA, Klassen DR, Feldman LS, et al. Evaluating laparoscopic skills: setting the pass/fail score for the MISTELS system. Surg Endosc 2003;17(6):964–7.
36. Vassiliou MC, Ghitulescu GA, Feldman LS, et al. The MISTELS program to measure technical skill in laparoscopic surgery: evidence for reliability. Surg Endosc 2006;20(5):744–7.
37. Black M, Gould JC. Measuring laparoscopic operative skill in a video trainer. Surg Endosc 2006;20(7):1069–71.
38. Adrales CL, Chu UB, Witzke DB, et al. Evaluating minimally invasive surgery training using low-cost mechanical simulations. Surg Endosc 2003;17:580–5.
39. Fried GM, Derossis AM, Bothwell J, et al. Comparison of laparoscopic performance in vivo with performance measured in a laparoscopic simulator. Surg Endosc 1999;13(11):1077–81.

40. Derossis AM, Antoniuk M, Fried GM. Evaluation of laparoscopic skills: a 2-year follow-up during residency training. Can J Surg 1999;42(4):293–7.
41. Peters JH, Fried GM, Swanstrom LL, et al. Development and validation of a comprehensive program of education and assessment of the basic fundamentals of laparoscopic surgery. Surgery 2004;135(1):21–7.
42. Fundamentals of laparoscopic surgery. Available at: http://www.flsprogram.org/. Accessed September 23, 2009.
43. ABS to require ACLS, ATLS and FLS for general surgery certification. Available at: http://home.absurgery.org/default.jsp?news_newreqs. Accessed October 28, 2009.
44. Soper NJ, Fried GM. The fundamentals of laparoscopic surgery: its time has come. Bull Am Coll Surg 2009;93(9):30–2.
45. Okrainec A, Smith L, Azzie G. Surgical simulation in Africa: the feasibility and impact of a 3-day fundamentals of laparoscopic surgery course. Surg Endosc 2009;23(11):2493–8.
46. Neary PC, Boyle E, Delaney CP, et al. Construct validation of a novel hybrid virtual-reality simulator for training and assessing laparoscopic colectomy; results from the first course for experienced senior laparoscopic surgeons. Surg Endosc 2008;22(10):2301–9.
47. Datta V, Mackay S, Mandalia M, et al. The use of electromagnetic motion tracking analysis to objectively measure open surgical skill in the laboratory-based model. J Am Coll Surg 2001;193(5):479–85.
48. Datta V, Chang A, Mackay S, et al. The relationship between motion analysis and surgical technical assessments. Am J Surg 2002;184(1):70–3.
49. Kuppersmith RB, Johnston R, Jones SB, et al. Virtual reality surgical simulation and otolaryngology. Arch Otolaryngol Head Neck Surg 1996;122(12):1297–8.
50. Satava RM. Virtual reality surgical simulator. Surg Endosc 1993;7:203–5.
51. Gurusamy KS, Aggarwal R, Palanivelu L, et al. Virtual reality training for surgical trainees in laparoscopic surgery [review] [104 refs]. Cochrane Database Syst Rev 2009;1:CD006575. DOI:10.1002/14651858.CD006575.pub2.
52. Seymour NE, Gallagher AG, Roman SA, et al. Virtual reality training improves operating room performance: results of a randomized, double-blinded study. Ann Surg 2002;236(4):458–64.
53. Grantcharov TP, Kristiansen VB, Bendix J, et al. Randomized clinical trial of virtual reality simulation for laparoscopic skills training. Br J Surg 2004;91:146–50.
54. Kothari SK, Kaplan BJ, DeMaria EJ, et al. Training in laparoscopic suturing skills using a new computer-based virtual reality simulator (MIST-VR) provides results comparable to those with an established pelvic trainer system. J Laparoendosc Adv Surg Tech A 2002;12(3):167–73.
55. Torkington J, Smith SGT, Rees BI, et al. Skill transfer from virtual reality to a real laparoscopic task. Surg Endosc 2001;15:1076–9.
56. Gallagher A, Richie K, McClure N, et al. Objective psychomotor skills assessment of experienced, junior, and novice laparoscopists with virtual reality. World J Surg 2001;25(11):1478–83.
57. Botden SM, Torab F, Buzink SN, et al. The importance of haptic feedback in laparoscopic suturing training and the additive value of virtual reality simulation. Surg Endosc 2008;22(5):1214–22.
58. Cao CG, Zhou M, Jones DB, et al. Can surgeons think and operate with haptics at the same time? J Gastrointest Surg 2007;11(11):1564–9.
59. Sutherland LM, Middleton PF, Anthony A, et al. Surgical simulation: a systematic review. Ann Surg 2006;243(3):291–300.

60. Woodrum DT, Andreatta PB, Yellamanchilli RK, et al. Construct validity of the LapSim laparoscopic surgical simulator. Am J Surg 2006;191(1):28–32.
61. KWv Dongen, Tournoij E, DCvd Zee, et al. Construct validity of the LapSim: Can the LapSim virtual reality simulator distinguish between novices and experts? Surg Endosc 2007;21:1413–7.
62. McDougall EM, Corica FA, Boker JR, et al. Construct validity testing of a laparoscopic surgical simulator. J Am Coll Surg 2006;202(5):779–87.
63. Andreatta PB, Woodrum DT, Gauger PG, et al. LapMentor metrics possess limited construct validity. Simul Healthc 2008;3:16–25.
64. Aggarwal R, Ward J, Balasundaram I, et al. Proving the effectiveness of virtual reality simulation for training in laparoscopic surgery. Ann Surg 2007;246:771–9.
65. Ahlberg G, Enochsson L, Gallagher AG, et al. Proficiency-based virtual reality training significantly reduces the error rate for residents during their first 10 laparoscopic cholecystectomies. Am J Surg 2009;193:797–804.
66. Andreatta PB, Woodrum DT, Birkmeyer JD, et al. Laparoscopic skills are improved with LapMentor training. Ann Surg 2006;243:854–63.
67. Nestel DF, Black SA, Kneebone RL, et al. Simulated anaesthetists in high fidelity simulations for surgical training: feasibility of a training programme for actors. Med Teach 2008;30(4):407–13.
68. Paige JT, Kozmenko V, Yang T, et al. Attitudinal changes resulting from repetitive training of operating room personnel using of high-fidelity simulation at the point of care. Am Surg 2009;75(7):584–90.
69. Powers KA, Rehrig ST, Irias N, et al. Simulated laparoscopic operating room crisis: An approach to enhance the surgical team performance. Surg Endosc 2008;22(4):885–900.
70. Perretta S, Dallemagne B, Coumaros D, et al. Natural orifice transluminal endoscopic surgery: transgastric cholecystectomy in a survival porcine model. Surg Endosc 2008;22(4):1126–30.
71. Hagen M, Wagner O, Swain P, et al. Hybrid natural orifice transluminal endoscopic surgery (NOTES) for Roux-en-Y gastric bypass: an experimental surgical study in human cadavers. Endoscopy 2008;40(11):918–24.
72. Spaun GO, Zheng B, Martinec DV, et al. Bimanual coordination in natural orifice transluminal endoscopic surgery: comparing the conventional dual-channel endoscope, the R-Scope, and a novel direct-drive system. Gastrointest Endosc 2009;69(6):39–45.
73. Gillen S, Wilhelm D, Meining A, et al. The "ELITE" model construct validation of a new training system for natural orifice transluminal endoscopic surgery (NOTES). Endoscopy 2009;41:395–9.
74. Gambadauro P, Magos A. NEST (network enhanced surgical training): a PC-based system for telementoring in gynaecological surgery. Eur J Obstet Gynecol Reprod Biol 2008;139(2):222–5.
75. Schlachta C, Lefebvre K, Sorsdahl A, et al. Mentoring and telementoring leads to effective incorporation of laparoscopic colon surgery. Surg Endosc 2009. [Epub ahead of print].
76. Sebajang H, Trudeau P, Dougall A, et al. Telementoring: an important enabling tool for the community surgeon. Surg Innov 2005;12(4):327–31.
77. Okrainec A, Henao O, Azzie G. Telesimulation: an effective method for teaching the fundamentals of laparoscopic surgery in resource-restricted countries. Surg Endosc 2009;24(2):417–22.

Optimal Acquisition and Assessment of Proficiency on Simulators in Surgery

Dimitrios Stefanidis, MD, PhD[a,b,*]

KEYWORDS

- Skills proficiency • Skills training • Simulators
- Performance assessment • Automaticity

The Halstedian apprenticeship model has governed surgical training for the last century.[1] Nevertheless, this model of training, also known as the "see one, do one, teach one" method has several limitations and is becoming obsolete today.

Many factors have been the impetus behind the recent paradigm shift in surgical residents' learning experiences, including concerns for patient safety, limited resident work hours, ethical concerns for learning new procedures on patients, pressures on teaching faculty for increased productivity and improved efficiency, the cost of resident training in the operating room, and the need for a more objective assessment of trainee skill in an era that has seen an exponential increase in new technology and procedures.[2]

The sole availability of a simulator, however, is not adequate to offer a meaningful educational experience to learners because the effectiveness of any simulator-based educational program is mainly dependent on the quality of its curriculum rather than on the tools (simulators) used.[3,4] It is the curriculum that brings life to the simulators and ensures learning. Nonetheless, to design appropriate skills curricula several considerations need to be taken into account, and a good understanding of how manual skills are best acquired is needed. Furthermore, it is imperative to understand the best ways to measure performance on simulators because this not only influences assessment but also has a profound impact on learning and the effectiveness of the skills curricula.

The aim of this article is to address the application of motor learning theory to simulator training, to highlight the important curricular elements for optimal skill acquisition,

Dr Stefanidis has no financial or personal relationships with people, products, or organizations that could inappropriately bias this work. No financial support was received for this work.
[a] Department of Surgery, University of North Carolina, Charlotte, NC, USA
[b] Carolinas Simulation Center and Division of Gastrointestinal and Minimally Invasive Surgery, Carolinas Medical Center, 1000 Blythe Boulevard, MEB 601, Charlotte, NC 28203, USA
* Carolinas Simulation Center and Division of Gastrointestinal and Minimally Invasive Surgery, Carolinas Medical Center, 1000 Blythe Boulevard, MEB 601, Charlotte, NC 28203, USA.
E-mail address: Dimitrios.Stefanidis@Carolinashealthcare.org

Surg Clin N Am 90 (2010) 475–489
doi:10.1016/j.suc.2010.02.010
0039-6109/10/$ – see front matter © 2010 Elsevier Inc. All rights reserved.

and to explore the best methods of performance assessment on simulators that maximize learning and skill transfer to the clinical environment.

MOTOR LEARNING THEORIES

According to Fitts and Posner,[5] complex manual skills are acquired in three sequential stages: a cognitive stage, an associative stage, and an autonomous stage. The application of this theory on surgical skill acquisition has been outlined nicely by Reznick and McCrae[2] who used the knot-tying task as an example. In the cognitive phase, surgical trainees read about and watch demonstrations of knot tying to understand the mechanics of the task. Without a clear understanding of the task at hand, it is impossible to proceed to the next level of learning. During the associative stage, trainees translate their knowledge into task performance by associating cognitive elements with musculoskeletal maneuvers and sensory input from their hands. Performance is initially erratic, but with practice, movements become smoother and more efficient leading to a series of well-coordinated movements. Finally, trainees reach the autonomous stage where psychomotor movements become automated with minimal demands on their attentional resources, which can be used for additional tasks, such as having a conversation.[2] Learning progresses sequentially through all these stages for every trainee, but the rate of progression may vary considerably and arrival at the last stage of learning can take a significant amount of time, which is dependent on the complexity of the learned task and the abilities of each trainee.[6]

Specific to simulators, several other curricular models closely resembling Fitts' three-stage progression have been proposed.[3,7–9] Gallagher and colleagues[7] describe eight steps important to all surgical skills curricula regardless of specialty or program:

1. Provide didactic teaching of relevant knowledge (ie, anatomy, pathology, physiology).
2. Provide instruction on the steps of the task or procedure.
3. Define and illustrate common errors.
4. Test all previous didactic information to ensure the student understands all the cognitive skills before going to the technical skills training, and in particular, to be able to determine when the student makes an error.
5. Provide technical skills training on the simulator.
6. Provide immediate (proximate) feedback when an error occurs.
7. Provide summative (terminal) feedback when an error occurs.
8. Iterate the skills training (repeated trials) while providing evidence at the end of each trial of progress (graphing the learning curve), with reference to a proficiency performance goal that the trainee is expected to attain.

McClusky and Smith[9] also propose a sequential, progressive, modular approach to curriculum development. In the first step, the cognitive elements of the task or procedure in question are taught using the appropriate resources. After the acquisition of the needed cognitive skills set, the innate abilities of trainees are tested, and simulator-based training follows to help translate cognition into motor behavior. Training occurs initially with instructors that provide performance feedback and continues with independent practice until a predefined set of proficiency criteria is reached. This progression continues for a series of tasks of increasing complexity until the simulator-based phase of the curriculum is completed. During this phase, trainees transition from the associative to the autonomous stage of learning. After performance benchmarks have been achieved in the skills lab, trainees transition to the real environment (operating room or wards) where they gain experience with patients and perfect their skills. The completion of this stage of training leads to the transition to independent application with the goal of maintenance of proficiency and skills mastery over months to years and throughout the surgeon's career (lifelong learning).[9]

Similarly, Aggarwal and colleagues[8] propose a competency-based framework for systematic training and assessment of technical skills. According to this framework, technical-skills learning begins with the acquisition of procedure-specific knowledge. Only after this knowledge is verified through testing, technical training begins. In addition, the task to be taught is deconstructed in its key components to facilitate learning, video recordings of the procedures are provided to trainees, and the tools for objective performance assessment are defined. Training models are then developed for the task in question and validated. Proficiency-based training on these validated models are then employed in the skills laboratory and the acquired skills are transferred to the real environment. The framework also maintains continuity of objective assessment in the real environment, using similar modes as in the skills laboratory. Through use of assessment tools in the real environment, participants in such a program can then be granted certification for independent practice of a technical procedure.

FACTORS AFFECTING THE EFFECTIVENESS OF THE CURRICULUM

The aforementioned theories provide a framework for curricular development on simulators. Nevertheless, several factors may impact the effectiveness of skills curricula and should be given consideration when designing them to optimize skill acquisition and transfer.

Deliberate Practice and Learner Motivation

Deliberate practice is essential for the acquisition of skills. Deliberate practice refers to a form of training that consists of focused, grueling, repetitive practice in which the learner continuously monitors his/her performance and subsequently corrects, experiments, and reacts to immediate and constant feedback, with the aim of steady and consistent improvement.[10,11] To engage in deliberate practice, learners need to be motivated internally, externally, or both. Although internal motivation is the most important driving force for learning, it is unique to each learner and difficult to modify by an external intervention. On the other hand, external motivation describes the interventions aimed at modifying behavior and may effectively produce the desired outcome. Thus, factors that impact learner motivation positively should be sought and incorporated into skills training, but caution should be exercised when doing so because learner motivation can also be impacted negatively. Examples of positive external-motivating factors during simulator training include providing learners with dedicated and protected practice time away from other responsibilities, encouraging healthy competition among residents by setting performance goals for them to reach and making the best performers known to the group, offering awards for their accomplishments, or setting requirements on simulators that need to be met before participation in the clinical environment is allowed. Mandatory participation in skills training may be the most effective motivator for residents who are subject to several negative external motivators that impact their participation, such as chronic fatigue, long working hours, limited free time, interference with clinical responsibilities, and accumulating operative experience that renders training on similar simulated tasks or procedures on inanimate models less stimulating. Empiric evidence from busy residency programs has demonstrated that resident participation in skills training was dismal (7%–14%) when the curriculum was voluntary, making the case for mandatory participation.[12,13]

Performance Feedback

For manual skills, feedback refers to the return of performance-related information to the performer and consists of intrinsic and extrinsic or augmented feedback.[14] Intrinsic feedback consists of performance-related information available directly to the sensory system of the performer (ie, the visual, auditory, or haptic perceptions during the performance of a task).[14] Research on simulators has indicated that interventions that enhance the internal feedback of the performer may improve skill acquisition. One example of such an intervention is the incorporation of haptic feedback to simulators. In a randomized crossover study, the provision of haptic feedback during the performance of a diathermy task led to improved performance compared with training without haptic feedback.[15] Other studies corroborate these findings,[16,17] but a recent review of the available evidence on the impact of haptic feedback on simulator skill acquisition concluded that even though the addition of haptic feedback appears beneficial, especially for the early phase of virtual reality training, the results were ambivalent and further study was needed in this area.[18]

Extrinsic or augmented feedback is performance-related information that is provided to the performer by an external source and aims to augment intrinsic feedback and lead to performance improvement. Augmented feedback facilitates the achievement of a skill and motivates the learner to continue putting effort toward the achievement of this skill,[14] thus aiding the skill-learning process. In medical education, such feedback to learners has been defined as an informed, non-evaluative appraisal of performance by the teacher.[19] Its purpose is to reinforce strengths and foster improvements in the learner by providing insight into actions and consequences and by highlighting the differences between the intended and the actual results of their actions.[19] The importance of augmented feedback for skill acquisition on simulators has been highlighted by several authors.[20–27] Several of these studies provide level I evidence, which clearly demonstrates that the provision of augmented feedback during simulator training versus no feedback at all results in improved skill acquisition and retention independent of the task in question. Although augmented feedback undoubtedly is essential for skill acquisition, its quality and the timing and frequency of its provision are of paramount importance. Augmented feedback can be provided to learners in a concurrent (during the performance of the task) or a summative (at the end of the task performance) fashion. In addition, the frequency and duration of either type of feedback can vary, possibly influencing performance. Winstein and Schmidt[28] first suggested in 1990 that the optimal frequency for providing augmented feedback is less than 100%. A recent study on simulators demonstrated this effect; intense, concurrent augmented feedback impaired acquisition of laparoscopic suturing skill compared with limited intermittent feedback provided after task completion.[26] Additional evidence provides support for improved learning when feedback is provided in a summative rather than concurrent fashion.[20,29] Accordingly, in a randomized, controlled trial by Xeroulis and colleagues, summary expert feedback after training sessions resulted in better skill retention compared with concurrent feedback for a suturing and knot-tying task.[20] The guidance hypothesis proposed by Winstein and Schmidt[28] provides a plausible explanation for these findings. According to this hypothesis, if augmented feedback is provided too frequently, it can cause the learner to develop dependency on its availability and to perform poorly in its absence. Thus, it is imperative that learners have practice time without feedback to develop their own learning strategies that can then be enhanced by appropriately timed, good-quality feedback. Nevertheless, although a reduced feedback frequency appears to benefit skill acquisition on simulators, the optimal frequency is unknown and task specific;

these areas need further study. In addition, little is known about appropriate delivery methods of performance feedback and the optimal training methods for instructors who provide such feedback.

Task Demonstration

Besides feedback, instruction and demonstration play a crucial role for motor skill training.[14,30] Effective instruction allows learners to understand the intricacies of a given task and assists them in forming a mental model for how to accomplish it. Among several instruction methods, the use of video tutorials is gaining popularity across disciplines. [14,31,32] Video-based education has proved effective for the acquisition of surgical skills on simulators.[33–36] Rosser and colleagues[34] demonstrated that a CD-ROM tutorial on laparoscopic skills effectively transferred the cognitive information necessary for skill development. In a further study from that group, trainees who watched a CD-ROM tutorial on laparoscopic suturing performed this task better compared with those who did not watch it.[25] More recently, Stefanidis and colleagues[26] demonstrated that frequent video-tutorial viewings during simulator training were associated with faster achievement of proficiency, and Xeroulis and colleagues[20] demonstrated that computer-based video instruction was as effective as expert feedback for the retention of simulator-acquired suturing and knot-tying skill. It should also be noted, that video tutorials provided before and during training are superior to those just provided before.[14]

Practice Distribution

Skill acquisition is also influenced by practice distribution. Distributed practice refers to learning a task in several training sessions with a period of rest between them, whereas during massed practice all training occurs in one session. Distributed practice is superior to massed practice for a variety of skills, but the size of this effect appears to be task dependent and influenced by the interval between training sessions (inter-training interval).[37–41] Still, some studies have demonstrated opposing findings.[42] For surgical skill acquisition, Moulton and colleagues[39] have confirmed in a randomized, controlled trial that residents retain and transfer microvascular anastomotic skill better if taught in a distributed rather than massed manner. The beneficial effect of distributed practice on skill acquisition is thought to be a consequence of the learning that occurs during rest periods between training sessions. According to a prior study by Karni and colleagues,[43] practice can set in motion neural processes that continue to evolve many hours after practice has ended. Thus, even a limited training experience can induce behaviorally significant changes in brain activity and initiate important long-term effects that may provide the basis for the consolidation of the initial learning experience.

Nevertheless, in a meta-analysis by Donovan and Radosevich[44] that examined the effect of practice distribution on performance, skill acquisition was improved when the inter-training interval was shorter, a finding that opposes the aforementioned theory. When the authors of this meta-analysis also included the type of task in their analysis, however, they noted that simple tasks were better acquired with shorter inter-training intervals, whereas more complex tasks required longer intervals.[44] A study that examined the effect of inter-training interval on surgical skill acquisition had similar findings; a basic laparoscopic task (fundamentals of laparoscopic surgery [FLS]-task 1: peg transfer) was acquired quicker by trainees who practiced every day compared with a group that practiced every week, but this was not true for a complex laparoscopic task (fundamentals of laparoscopic surgery [FLS]-task 5: intracorporeal suturing) where there were no significant differences between the two groups in skill acquisition rate.[45]

Because the impact of practice distribution and inter-training interval on skill acquisition is task specific, additional study is needed to identify the optimal training sequence for various surgical skills. In addition, the optimal duration of each training session should be reexamined because, at the present time, it is chosen arbitrarily.

Task Difficulty and Practice Variability

The literature suggests that skill acquisition is influenced by practice variability and training under increasing levels of difficulty.[46–49] A systematic review regarding the effect of high-fidelity medical simulations on learning found that learning was enhanced when trainees had the opportunity to practice with progressively increasing levels of difficulty.[46] In addition, using the minimally invasive surgical trainer-virtual reality (Mentice Inc, Evanston, IL, USA) simulator, Ali and colleagues[50] demonstrated that training on the medium level resulted in improved skill acquisition when compared with training on the easy level. Progressively increasing levels of difficulty has also been suggested to be optimal for curriculum design.[51] Training in a complex laparoscopic task under more difficult conditions has also been demonstrated to lead to performance improvements on a simulator, but had limited impact on the transfer of the acquired skill to the operating room.[49]

Contextual interference refers to the learning effectiveness of random versus blocked practice.[52] Several studies have suggested that learning is enhanced when different tasks are practiced randomly rather than in a specific order (blocked practice) and when training incorporates practice variability.[52–56] Nevertheless, this effect is not consistent and appears to be dependent on task complexity and other factors.[47,57]

Proficiency-based Training

Proficiency-based simulator training leads to improved operative performance and is considered by many experts the ideal training paradigm on simulators.[58–61] Proficiency-based curricula set training goals that are derived from expert performance and give learners a performance target to achieve. By providing such performance targets and immediate performance feedback to learners via knowledge of results (at the end of each repetition learners can compare their performance to these targets), this type of training promotes deliberate practice, boosts motivation, and enhances skill acquisition.[14,62] Indeed, a recent study demonstrated that setting performance goals on simulators boosted resident attendance and participation in the skills laboratory.[62] Furthermore, proficiency-based curricula tailor training to individual learner needs and produce uniform skill, because training is considered complete when the same objective performance goals have been achieved by all learners.

In contrast, traditional training paradigms, such as time-based curricula, set a specified training duration, whereas repetition-based curricula set a minimum number of repetitions on the required tasks before training is considered complete. The main limitations of these curricula are that they do not take into account individual learning differences and often use arbitrary training endpoints (number of hours or repetitions). Given that learners have different baseline abilities, prior experiences, and motivation that impact skill acquisition, such curricula can lead to inadequate training or overtraining. The superiority of proficiency-based over duration- or repetition-based training has been highlighted by several experts in the field[4,7,51,63] and is obvious from the example in **Fig. 1**. In addition, by not having a defined training goal, learner efforts might be misdirected and their motivation to practice negatively affected, further impacting eventual performance. Empiric evidence supports the superiority of proficiency-based training.

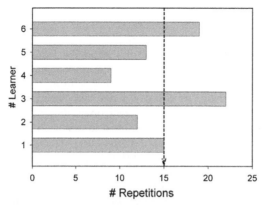

Fig. 1. Figure illustrating the superiority of proficiency-based curricula over time or repetition-based curricula. Bars represent the number of repetitions it took each learner to achieve expert derived performance levels (proficiency) on a task. If training duration would be set at 15 repetitions of the task, learners 3 and 6 would have received inadequate training, whereas learners 2,4, and 5 would have trained too long to achieve the same level of performance.

In a randomized trial, Madan and colleagues[64] demonstrated that residents who were given a goal for training on eight simulated laparoscopic tasks outperformed those who practiced for equal amounts of time but without goals. Brydges and colleagues[65] demonstrated in a randomized, controlled trial that self-guided training with process goals (where participants set goals focused on performance mechanisms) was more effective in imparting wound-closure skills to medical students compared with self-guided training with outcome goals (where participants set goals focused on performance products) indicating that the way training goals are defined may also be important for skill acquisition.

This study brings forward one of the important issues when using goal-directed training, which is how to define such goals. In the proficiency-based training paradigm, such goals are based on expert-derived performance. Because the intention of training inexperienced learners is to help them shape their performance to mimic experts, deriving training goals from expert performance appears intuitive. Yet, this approach is inherently flawed by our poor understanding of surgical expertise,[10,66] which introduces arbitrary choice to the methods we use to define simulator proficiency.

PERFORMANCE ASSESSMENT

According to Ericsson,[10] who has studied expertise extensively, expertise is domain- and task-specific and is achieved by deliberate practice over several years. Experts show maximal adaptation to task constraints and have consistency in their performance.[11] Still, many questions need to be answered using high-quality evidence. For example, how should expertise in surgery be defined and measured? What is the most appropriate way to establish proficiency levels based on expert performance? How should expertise be detected when it is achieved on simulators by learners? Should expert levels be used as simulation-based training endpoints or might less difficult performance levels be more appropriate? Nevertheless, without accurate and appropriate metrics for identifying superior performance, it is impossible to find an adequate answer to most of these questions.

Traditionally, the easily obtainable metrics of task duration and errors have been used for performance assessment during skills curricula. Learners practice repetitively until they reach a more efficient and error-free performance. Unfortunately, such metrics do not provide insight regarding the effort the individual had to invest to achieve a specific level of performance, or whether learning has been completed.[67,68] Thus, task duration and errors may not be the most appropriate performance metrics for proficiency-based training. As a result, when only time and errors are used to establish proficiency criteria for simulator training goals, they may provide a misleading picture of a trainee's level of skill and readiness to transition to the clinical environment. Indeed, several prior studies have demonstrated that although surgical trainees are able to achieve expert-level performance based on time and error metrics on simulators, their performance falls short of true expert skill in the more demanding and stressful conditions of the operating room.[49,58,61] This finding could be related to the inadequacy of the traditional metrics to assess when simulator learning is complete. Thus, additional, more sensitive performance metrics, such as limb kinematics (trajectory, velocity, and acceleration); global rating scales; psychophysiologic measures (electromyography, EEG, and so forth); and measures of mental workload,[67,68] may provide complementary performance assessment that may augment skill acquisition and transfer.

Observer Ratings

Besides using the traditional metrics of time and errors, surgical performance can also be reliably assessed by an experienced observer. In fact, this type of assessment is preferable for some skills as it provides qualitative information on learner performance that can then be provided as summative and formative feedback to the learner.[69,70] Furthermore, these instruments are versatile as they can often be used for similar tasks. Because by definition this type of assessment relies on subjective ratings, it is imperative that the reliability and validity of such instruments be proved before their use for evaluation.[69] Instruments typically used include global rating scales, visual analog scales, checklists, or a combination of these. Evidence suggests that global rating scales are superior to checklists, specifically for the evaluation of technical skill, when completed by experts.[71,72] Furthermore, checklists and visual analog scales have failed to enhance the effectiveness of performance assessment compared with global rating scales alone and should therefore not be included in this type of assessment.[69,72] Validated rating scales for technical skill assessment have been developed for open objective structured assessment of technical skill[70] and global operative assessment of laparoscopic skills[69] and should be incorporated in simulator training. Nevertheless, the exact relationship of this type of assessment with other more objective performance metrics is not well studied.

Automaticity

One of the main skilled-performer (expert) characteristics that distinguish them from novices is their ability to engage in certain activities without requiring significant attentional resources. To describe this characteristic, Shiffrin and Schneider first used the term automaticity.[73,74] Habitual or highly practiced motor acts can be performed automatically, leaving enough spare attentional capacity for engagement in multiple activities. In contrast to experts, novices who practice on a new and unfamiliar task are often operating at maximal attentional capacity, feel overwhelmed by the task, and are incapable of attending to other stimuli from their environment, which can impact safety. Attending surgeons are familiar with this phenomenon because sometimes it may be difficult to attract the attention of junior trainees who are performing procedures unfamiliar to them. For example, there may be a lag in a trainee's response to verbal cues by the attending. Automaticity has been used in the motor-skill literature to identify skilled performers and confirm learning by novices.[6,14,67,75–77] The attainment of automaticity has even been mapped to specific areas of the brain that differ from those used by novices unfamiliar with a particular task.[75] The best way to produce automaticity is through repeated practice on tasks with consistently mapped characteristics.[73] This type of practice is reflective of deliberate practice that, according to Ericsson, is the hallmark for the achievement of superior performance.[10,11] To measure automaticity and spare attentional capacity, the most common procedure used is that of a secondary task that must be performed concurrently with the primary task.[6,14,67,74–77] For example, if a trainee is learning how to suture (primary task), they would also have to perform a simultaneous secondary task that competes for the same attentional resources as the primary task. In this instance, measuring the performance on the secondary task reflects how much attention the learner can spare from the primary task to invest in the secondary task and thus, how comfortable they are with the performance of the primary task and how automated their performance is. Several tasks can be used as secondary tasks, but the secondary task must compete with the same attentional resources as the primary task to provide a sensitive measure of automaticity. As an example, if the primary task requires significant visual-spatial attentional resources, the secondary task should also draw from the same visual-spatial resources to provide the most sensitive assessment of learner automaticity; in contrast, a secondary task that uses auditory resources may be distracting but would not be as sensitive.

A previous study investigating this concept for laparoscopic suturing on a simulator found that trainees who achieved the same performance as experts according to time and errors metrics performed significantly worse according to a visual-spatial secondary task; this finding indicated that the latter was a more sensitive metric of expert performance.[67] A follow-up study also demonstrated that the training duration to achieve automaticity based on performance on a secondary task was far longer than the training interval required to reach proficiency based on the metrics of time and errors alone.[6] These findings were confirmed in a recent randomized, controlled trial where achievement of automaticity using a secondary-task metric was also accompanied by improved skill transfer to the operating room (Stefanidis and colleagues, unpublished data, 2010). Based on these findings, it becomes clear that although the traditional metrics of time and errors may be good performance measures during the early stages of learning, they provide a rather inadequate assessment of skilled performers. It is for the latter stages of learning where more sensitive performance metrics, such as the secondary-task approach, are needed.

Workload Assessment

For a more complete performance assessment, besides secondary-task metrics, other metrics may also be of importance. Learner performance may be influenced by task workload, performance anxiety, and stress. Task workload tends to be higher during the early stages of learning and decreases as learners become more experienced with the task. Indeed, a previous study that evaluated the performance of surgeons with different levels of experience on a camera-navigation task found that more skilled individuals experienced less workload when performing the task compared with less experienced individuals.[78] Importantly, increased workload during the performance of a task may increase operator fatigue and frustration and compromise attention span. As a consequence, when workload is high, the capacity to deal with new or unexpected task demands may be impaired, task routine may be disorganized, and the likelihood of performance errors may increase.[79] Prior studies have demonstrated that increased surgeon fatigue and mental demands during laparoscopy may increase the duration of the procedure and the number of errors made.[80–82] In a review, Young and colleagues[83] highlighted the importance of developing a method for measuring workload to prevent errors and provide safe and cost-effective care; these investigators recommended the National Aeronautics and Space Administration–Task Load Index (NASA-TLX) tool as a sensitive assessment instrument.

The NASA-TLX is a validated tool for workload self assessment that measures the mental, physical, and temporal demands of a task and the effort, frustration, and perceived performance of the trainee on a 20-point visual analog scale.[84] This tool helps quantify task-specific individual workload components and has been validated and employed initially by the Human Performance Group at the NASA Ames Research Laboratory as a tool for subjective evaluation of an individual's workload during flight simulation. More recently, it has been widely used in a variety of tasks outside of the aeronautic field for assessment of workload perception,[49,78,79,85,86] and is sufficiently sensitive to produce meaningful data on workload assessment.[85] The NASA-TLX workload scores also mirror performance changes as measured using the traditional metrics of time and errors during simulator training.[49] Thus, mounting evidence suggests that the NASA-TLX workload-assessment tool provides a reliable measure of workload, task difficulty, and learner comfort with a task during simulator training and during transition to the operating room. Because workload significantly impacts performance and the NASA-TLX tool is easily obtainable, accurately measures workload, and provides performance information not otherwise available to the learner or the trainer, it should be incorporated as an additional metric during simulator training and for surgical skill assessment in general.

Performance Anxiety and Physiologic Measures of Performance

Mental strain or stress has been implicated previously as one possible factor for technical errors or inferior performance by the primary surgeon,[82] perhaps even more so for minimally invasive surgery than for conventional surgery.[81,82] Because stress may be difficult to evaluate or to quantify with subjective measures, physiologic measures, such as heart rate variability, have been used previously as more objective indicators of stress.[87,88] Indeed, studies from the field of aviation have concluded that heart-rate recordings are the most useful psychophysiologic variables[87,89] to assess pilot's workload and mental strain and are likely superior to and less biased than subjective reporting. Moreover, Mongin and colleagues[90] found a 4% to 10% increase in the heart rate of surgical trainees during the performance of laparoscopic cholecystectomy. Furthermore, Bohm and colleagues[91] studied the heart rate of experienced surgeons during colorectal surgery and found that a laparoscopic approach or being the operating surgeon was associated with increased stress compared with an open approach or being the assistant surgeon. In a recent study, Prabhu and colleagues found evidence that linked incomplete operating room transferability of simulator-acquired skills with a significant increase in the trainee's heart rate in the operating room compared with the simulator.[92] Thus, physiologic measures may also provide complementary information on learner performance not otherwise available; these metrics should also be considered during simulator training.

SUMMARY

The theoretical framework behind surgical skill acquisition supports factors that can optimize skills curricula and trainee learning, such that learner proficiency may be ultimately achieved. The available evidence for the best performance-assessment methods suggests that the incorporation of additional, more sensitive performance metrics may lead to improved skill transfer. Simulator curricula that take into account the aforementioned factors can optimize skill acquisition and lead to improved learner readiness for the operating room.

REFERENCES

1. Osborne MP. William Stewart Halsted: his life and contributions to surgery. Lancet Oncol 2007;8(3):256–65.
2. Reznick RK, MacRae H. Teaching surgical skills–changes in the wind. N Engl J Med 2006;355(25):2664–9.
3. Satava RM. Disruptive visions: surgical education. Surg Endosc 2004;18(5): 779–81.
4. Fried GM. Lessons from the surgical experience with simulators: incorporation into training and utilization in determining competency. Gastrointest Endosc Clin N Am 2006;16(3):425–34.
5. Fitts PM, Posner MI. Human performance. Belmont (CA): Brooks/Cole; 1967.
6. Stefanidis D, Scerbo MW, Sechrist C, et al. Do novices display automaticity during simulator training? Am J Surg 2008;195(2):210–3.
7. Gallagher AG, Ritter EM, Champion H, et al. Virtual reality simulation for the operating room: proficiency-based training as a paradigm shift in surgical skills training. Ann Surg 2005;241(2):364–72.
8. Aggarwal R, Grantcharov TP, Darzi A. Framework for systematic training and assessment of technical skills. J Am Coll Surg 2007;204(4):697–705.
9. McClusky DA 3rd, Smith CD. Design and development of a surgical skills simulation curriculum. World J Surg 2008;32(2):171–81.
10. Ericsson KA. Deliberate practice and the acquisition and maintenance of expert performance in medicine and related domains. Acad Med 2004;79(10 Suppl): S70–81.
11. Ericsson KA, Lehmann AC. Expert and exceptional performance: evidence of maximal adaptation to task constraints. Annu Rev Psychol 1996;47:273–305.
12. Chang L, Petros J, Hess DT, et al. Integrating simulation into a surgical residency program: is voluntary participation effective? Surg Endosc 2007;21(3):418–21.
13. Stefanidis D, Acker CE, Swiderski D, et al. Challenges during the implementation of a laparoscopic skills curriculum in a busy general surgery residency program. J Surg Educ 2008;65(1):4–7.
14. Magill RA. Motor learning and control. Concepts and applications. 7th edition. New York: McGraw-Hill; 2004.
15. Strom P, Hedman L, Sarna L, et al. Early exposure to haptic feedback enhances performance in surgical simulator training: a prospective randomized crossover study in surgical residents. Surg Endosc 2006;20(9):1383–8.
16. Cao CG, Zhou M, Jones DB, et al. Can surgeons think and operate with haptics at the same time? J Gastrointest Surg 2007;11(11):1564–9.
17. Panait L, Akkary E, Bell RL, et al. The role of haptic feedback in laparoscopic simulation training. J Surg Res 2009;156(2):312–6.
18. van der Meijden OA, Schijven MP. The value of haptic feedback in conventional and robot-assisted minimal invasive surgery and virtual reality training: a current review. Surg Endosc 2009;23(6):1180–90.
19. Ende J. Feedback in clinical medical education. JAMA 1983;250(6):777–81.

20. Xeroulis GJ, Park J, Moulton CA, et al. Teaching suturing and knot-tying skills to medical students: a randomized controlled study comparing computer-based video instruction and (concurrent and summary) expert feedback. Surgery 2007;141(4):442–9.

21. Porte MC, Xeroulis G, Reznick RK, et al. Verbal feedback from an expert is more effective than self-accessed feedback about motion efficiency in learning new surgical skills. Am J Surg 2007;193(1):105–10.

22. Mahmood T, Darzi A. The learning curve for a colonoscopy simulator in the absence of any feedback: no feedback, no learning. Surg Endosc 2004;18(8): 1224–30.

23. Chang JY, Chang GL, Chien CJ, et al. Effectiveness of two forms of feedback on training of a joint mobilization skill by using a joint translation simulator. Phys Ther 2007;87(4):418–30.

24. Kruglikova I, Grantcharov TP, Drewes AM, et al. The impact of constructive feedback on training in gastrointestinal endoscopy using high fidelity virtual reality simulation. A randomized controlled trial. Gut 2010;59(2):181–5.

25. Pearson AM, Gallagher AG, Rosser JC, et al. Evaluation of structured and quantitative training methods for teaching intracorporeal knot tying. Surg Endosc 2002;16(1):130–7.

26. Stefanidis D, Korndorffer JR Jr, Heniford BT, et al. Limited feedback and video tutorials optimize learning and resource utilization during laparoscopic simulator training. Surgery 2007;142(2):202–6.

27. Rogers DA, Regehr G, Howdieshell TR, et al. The impact of external feedback on computer-assisted learning for surgical technical skill training. Am J Surg 2000; 179(4):341–3.

28. Winstein CJ, Schmidt RA. Reduced frequency of knowledgeof results enhances motor skill learning. J Exp Psychol Learn Mem Cogn 1990;16:677–91.

29. Schmidt RA, Wulf G. Continuous concurrent feedback degrades skill learning: implications for training and simulation. Hum Factors 1997;39(4):509–25.

30. Hodges NJ, Franks IM. Modelling coaching practice: the role of instruction and demonstration. J Sports Sci 2002;20(10):793–811.

31. McGraw-Hunter M, Faw GD, Davis PK. The use of video self-modelling and feedback to teach cooking skills to individuals with traumatic brain injury: a pilot study. Brain Inj 2006;20(10):1061–8.

32. Scherer LA, Chang MC, Meredith JW, et al. Videotape review leads to rapid and sustained learning. Am J Surg 2003;185(6):516–20.

33. Jowett N, LeBlanc V, Xeroulis G, et al. Surgical skill acquisition with self-directed practice using computer-based video training. Am J Surg 2007;193(2):237–42.

34. Rosser JC, Herman B, Risucci DA, et al. Effectiveness of a CD-ROM multimedia tutorial in transferring cognitive knowledge essential for laparoscopic skill training. Am J Surg 2000;179(4):320–4.

35. Takiguchi S, Sekimoto M, Yasui M, et al. Cyber visual training as a new method for the mastery of endoscopic surgery. Surg Endosc 2005;19(9):1204–10.

36. Summers AN, Rinehart GC, Simpson D, et al. Acquisition of surgical skills: a randomized trial of didactic, videotape, and computer-based training. Surgery 1999;126(2):330–6.

37. Dail TK, Christina RW. Distribution of practice and metacognition in learning and long-term retention of a discrete motor task. Res Q Exerc Sport 2004;75(2):148–55.

38. Lee T, Genovese E. Distribution of practice in motor skill acquisition: learning and performance effects reconsidered. Res Q 1988;59:277–87.

39. Moulton CA, Dubrowski A, Macrae H, et al. Teaching surgical skills: what kind of practice makes perfect?: a randomized, controlled trial. Ann Surg 2006;244(3): 400–9.

40. Lee TD, Genovese ED. Distribution of practice in motor skill acquisition: different effects for discrete and continuous tasks. Res Q Exerc Sport 1989;60(1):59–65.

41. Mackay S, Morgan P, Datta V, et al. Practice distribution in procedural skills training: a randomized controlled trial. Surg Endosc 2002;16(6):957–61.

42. Garcia JA, Moreno FJ, Reina R, et al. Analysis of effects of distribution of practice in learning and retention of a continuous and a discrete skill presented on a computer. Percept Mot Skills 2008;107(1):261–72.

43. Karni A, Meyer G, Rey-Hipolito C, et al. The acquisition of skilled motor performance: fast and slow experience-driven changes in primary motor cortex. Proc Natl Acad Sci U S A 1998;95(3):861–8.

44. Donovan J, Radosevich DJ. A meta-analytic review of the distribution of practice effect: now you see it, now you don't. J Appl Psychol 1999;84(5):795–805.

45. Zoog E, Acker CE, Swiderski D, et al. Do shorter training intervals lead to superior skill acquisition during proficiency-based simulator training? J Am Coll Surg 2009;209(3):S109.

46. Issenberg SB, McGaghie WC, Petrusa ER, et al. Features and uses of high-fidelity medical simulations that lead to effective learning: a BEME systematic review. Med Teach 2005;27(1):10–28.

47. Hall KG, Magill RA. Variability of practice and contextual interference in motor skill learning. J Mot Behav 1995;27(4):299–309.

48. Giuffrida CG, Shea JB, Fairbrother JT. Differential transfer benefits of increased practice for constant, blocked, and serial practice schedules. J Mot Behav 2002;34(4):353–65.

49. Stefanidis D, Korndorffer JR Jr, Markley S, et al. Closing the gap in operative performance between novices and experts: does harder mean better for laparoscopic simulator training? J Am Coll Surg 2007;205(2):307–13.

50. Ali MR, Mowery Y, Kaplan B, et al. Training the novice in laparoscopy. More challenge is better. Surg Endosc 2002;16(12):1732–6.

51. Aggarwal R, Grantcharov T, Moorthy K, et al. A competency-based virtual reality training curriculum for the acquisition of laparoscopic psychomotor skill. Am J Surg 2006;191(1):128–33.

52. Wulf G, Lee TD. Contextual interference in movements of the same class: differential effects on program and parameter learning. J Mot Behav 1993;25(4): 254–63.

53. Jarus T, Wughalter EH, Gianutsos JG. Effects of contextual interference and conditions of movement task on acquisition, retention, and transfer of motor skills by women. Percept Mot Skills 1997;84(1):179–93.

54. Proteau L, Blandin Y, Alain C, et al. The effects of the amount and variability of practice on the learning of a multi-segmented motor task. Acta Psychol (Amst) 1994;85(1):61–74.

55. Bortoli L, Robazza C, Durigon V, et al. Effects of contextual interference on learning technical sports skills. Percept Mot Skills 1992;75(2):555–62.

56. Kurahashi A, Leming K, Carnahan H, et al. Effects of expertise, practice and contextual interference on adaptations to visuo-motor misalignment. Stud Health Technol Inform 2008;132:225–9.

57. Brady F. Contextual interference: a meta-analytic study. Percept Mot Skills 2004; 99(1):116–26.

58. Korndorffer JR Jr, Dunne JB, Sierra R, et al. Simulator training for laparoscopic suturing using performance goals translates to the operating room. J Am Coll Surg 2005;201(1):23–9.
59. Ahlberg G, Enochsson L, Gallagher AG, et al. Proficiency-based virtual reality training significantly reduces the error rate for residents during their first 10 laparoscopic cholecystectomies. Am J Surg 2007;193(6):797–804.
60. Seymour NE, Gallagher AG, Roman SA, et al. Virtual reality training improves operating room performance: results of a randomized, double-blinded study. Ann Surg 2002;236(4):458–63 [discussion: 463–4].
61. Stefanidis D, Acker C, Heniford BT. Proficiency-based laparoscopic simulator training leads to improved operating room skill that is resistant to decay. Surg Innov 2008;15(1):69–73.
62. Walters KC, Acker CE, Heniford BT, et al. Performance goals on simulators boost resident motivation and skills lab attendance. J Am Coll Surg 2008;207(3):S88.
63. Stefanidis D, Heniford BT. The formula for a successful laparoscopic skills curriculum. Arch Surg 2009;144(1):77–82 [discussion: 82].
64. Madan AK, Harper JL, Taddeucci RJ, et al. Goal-directed laparoscopic training leads to better laparoscopic skill acquisition. Surgery 2008;144(2):345–50.
65. Brydges R, Carnahan H, Safir O, et al. How effective is self-guided learning of clinical technical skills? It's all about process. Med Educ 2009;43(6):507–15.
66. Ericsson KA. Deliberate practice and acquisition of expert performance: a general overview. Acad Emerg Med 2008;15(11):988–94.
67. Stefanidis D, Scerbo MW, Korndorffer JR Jr, et al. Redefining simulator proficiency using automaticity theory. Am J Surg 2007;193(4):502–6.
68. O'Donnell RD, Eggemeier FT. Workload assessment methodology. In: Boff KR, Kaufman L, Thomas JP, editors. Handbook of perception and performance, Cognitive processes and performance, vol. 2. New York: Wiley; 1986. p. 1–49.
69. Vassiliou MC, Feldman LS, Andrew CG, et al. A global assessment tool for evaluation of intraoperative laparoscopic skills. Am J Surg 2005;190(1):107–13.
70. Martin JA, Regehr G, Reznick R, et al. Objective structured assessment of technical skill (OSATS) for surgical residents. Br J Surg 1997;84(2):273–8.
71. Regehr G, MacRae H, Reznick RK, et al. Comparing the psychometric properties of checklists and global rating scales for assessing performance on an OSCE-format examination. Acad Med 1998;73(9):993–7.
72. Hodges B, Regehr G, McNaughton N, et al. OSCE checklists do not capture increasing levels of expertise. Acad Med 1999;74(10):1129–34.
73. Shiffrin RM, Schneider W. Controlled and automatic human information processing: II. Perceptual learning, automatic attending, and a general theory. Psychol Rev 1977;84:127–90.
74. Logan GD. Automaticity, resources, and memory: theoretical controversies and practical implications. Hum Factors 1988;30(5):583–98.
75. Floyer-Lea A, Matthews PM. Changing brain networks for visuomotor control with increased movement automaticity. J Neurophysiol 2004;92(4):2405–12.
76. Wickens CD, Hollands JG. Engineering psychology and human performance. 3rd edition. Upper Saddle River (NJ): Prentice Hall; 2000.
77. Schmidt RA, Lee TD. Motor control and learning: a behavioral emphasis. Champain (IL): Human Kinetics Publishers; 2005.
78. Stefanidis D, Haluck R, Pham T, et al. Construct and face validity and task workload for laparoscopic camera navigation: virtual reality versus video trainer systems at the SAGES Learning Center. Surg Endosc 2007;21(7):1158–64.

79. Weinger MB, Herndon OW, Zornow MH, et al. An objective methodology for task analysis and workload assessment in anesthesia providers. Anesthesiology 1994;80(1):77–92.
80. Berguer R, Smith WD, Chung YH. Performing laparoscopic surgery is significantly more stressful for the surgeon than open surgery. Surg Endosc 2001; 15(10):1204–7.
81. Munch-Petersen HR, Rosenberg J. [Physical and mental strain on the surgeon during minimally invasive surgery]. Ugeskr Laeger 2008;170(8):624–9 [in Danish].
82. Schuetz M, Gockel I, Beardi J, et al. Three different types of surgeon-specific stress reactions identified by laparoscopic simulation in a virtual scenario. Surg Endosc 2008;22(5):1263–7.
83. Young G, Zavelina L, Hooper V. Assessment of workload using NASA Task Load Index in perianesthesia nursing. J Perianesth Nurs 2008;23(2):102–10.
84. Hart SG, Staveland LE. Development of NASA-TLX (task load index): Results of empirical and theoretical research. In: Hancock PA, Meshkati N, editors. Human mental workload. Amsterdam (The Netherlands): Elsevier; 1988. p. 139–83.
85. Weinger MB, Vredenburgh AG, Schumann CM, et al. Quantitative description of the workload associated with airway management procedures. J Clin Anesth 2000;12(4):273–82.
86. Stefanidis D, Wang F, Korndorffer JR Jr, et al. Robotic assistance improves intracorporeal suturing performance and safety in the operating room while decreasing operator workload. Surg Endosc 2010;24(2):377–82.
87. Roscoe AH. Assessing pilot workload. Why measure heart rate, HRV and respiration? Biol Psychol 1992;34(2–3):259–87.
88. Veltman JA, Gaillard AW. Physiological workload reactions to increasing levels of task difficulty. Ergonomics 1998;41(5):656–69.
89. Jorna PG. Heart rate and workload variations in actual and simulated flight. Ergonomics 1993;36(9):1043–54.
90. Mongin C, Dufour F, Lattanzio F, et al. [Evaluation of stress in surgical trainees: prospective study of heart rate during laparoscopic cholecystectomy]. J Chir (Paris) 2008;145(2):138–42 [in French].
91. Bohm B, Rotting N, Schwenk W, et al. A prospective randomized trial on heart rate variability of the surgical team during laparoscopic and conventional sigmoid resection. Arch Surg 2001;136(3):305–10.
92. Prabhu A, Smith W, Yurko YY, et al. Increased stress levels may explain the incomplete transfer of simulator-acquired skill to the operating room. Surgery 2010. [Epub ahead of print].

Running a Surgical Education Center: From Small to Large

Andreas H. Meier, MD[a,b,]*

KEYWORDS

• Surgical simulation • Skills • Education • Training

Ever since modern surgical training started with Dr Halsted's concept of a structured residency program more than 100 years ago,[1] the operating room (OR) has served as the education laboratory to develop expertise in technical skills. The "see one, do one, teach one" paradigm guided surgical educators and was successful in creating a highly skilled surgical workforce. This concept, however, depended on a large volume and high variety of cases.[2] Increasing concerns regarding patient safety,[3] shortening of the resident work hours,[4,5] and the developing economic pressures within health care affecting traditional resident teaching[6,7] resulted in further rethinking of the Halstedian system. The paradigm shift toward moving the learning curve outside of the OR, however, was not so much initiated by concerns regarding surgical residency training but caused by the need to train surgeons already in practice. This need became most obvious in the early 1990s with the advent of minimally invasive surgery. The challenge of safely introducing highly trained individuals to a novel, disruptive surgical technology resulted in a strong academic interest in skills training within the surgical specialties. At the same time, other medical disciplines had successfully demonstrated the concept of simulation in medical education.[8,9] Vast improvements in computer technology and virtual reality (VR) made the simulation of surgical tasks and procedures feasible. In 1999, the Accreditation Council for Graduate Medical Education (ACGME) embarked on its outcomes project, which ultimately required residency programs to demonstrate and measure clearly defined competencies in their trainees.[10] Some institutions recognized early on that surgical skills laboratories were ideally suited to assess technical skills in a controllable and safe environment.[11] Multiple studies have confirmed that transfer of skills from simulated environments to the real world occurs.[12,13]

At present, the concept of providing portions of the surgical curriculum outside of ORs and wards using simulation technology has become widely accepted within

a Surgical Skills Center, Southern Illinois University, PO Box 19665, Springfield, IL 62794, USA
b Division of Pediatric Surgery, Department of Surgery, Southern Illinois University, PO Box 19665, Springfield, IL 62794, USA
* Surgical Skills Center, Southern Illinois University, PO Box 19665, Springfield, IL 62794.
E-mail address: ameier@siumed.edu

Surg Clin N Am 90 (2010) 491–504
doi:10.1016/j.suc.2010.02.003
0039-6109/10/$ – see front matter © 2010 Elsevier Inc. All rights reserved.

the surgical community. This acceptance may be best reflected in the most recent Residency Review Committee (RRC) requirements for surgical training programs recommending access to "simulation and skills laboratories."[14]

Despite simulation and skills training becoming mainstream within surgical education, many institutions are still struggling with the successful integration of such programs. In 2004, 80% of the respondents of a survey of surgical residency programs stated that they had access to skills laboratories for laparoscopic surgery, but their use varied widely.[15] Even though many surgical programs refer to learning centers as a "skills lab," their educational concept can and should go beyond pure technical skills training. The facility's main objective should be to enrich the educational experience of medical students and residents, provide an environment for deliberate practice, and allow assessment and remediation of trainees in a safe setting.

This article outlines important general principles for the successful integration of surgical simulation and skills facilities into the surgical training programs and their curriculum. These principles apply to all such centers independent of their specific objectives and size.

BASIC PRINCIPLES FOR SUCCESS: SUPPORT, SPACE, AND PERSONNEL REQUIREMENTS

The successful implementation of a surgical simulation program is nearly impossible without the support of departmental leadership. The enthusiasm of the chairperson and surgical residency program director for skills training and simulation is of crucial importance to develop the educational culture within the department that is necessary to motivate the faculty and the trainees. It is not enough to just create a small skills laboratory in an effort to fulfill the RRC requirements. True success requires integration of simulation into the departmental curricula, which ensures the use of the laboratory by the trainees and calls for the participation of the faculty but depends on the support and resource allocation by the departmental leadership. Departmental buy-in is not always a given and is sometimes difficult to gain, as the return of investment for surgical education centers is hard to quantify in pure financial terms. Despite improving evidence for the validity of simulation in medical education,[16] such an argument alone may not be enough to convince the authorities. It is important to emphasize that traditional education within the clinical environment is even more expensive and inefficient[16] and, in addition, carries the potential risk of patient safety compromise and suboptimal quality of care. Recent studies showing that VR skills training shortens OR time[17] may ultimately provide enough of a financial incentive to increase support for such training.

Adequate space is an important prerequisite for the successful implementation of a surgical education laboratory. Before deciding on the square footage for the center, however, it is important to define the objectives for the facility and its overall scope. To accomplish this, at least 4 questions must be posed: Will this space be used solely for surgical skills training? Will the center include curricula for full patient simulator training? Will team training occur? Will this be a multidisciplinary facility? Space planning for the center should be based on these objectives. It is helpful for the stakeholders to visit established education centers with similar objectives elsewhere and learn from the experiences at these institutions. Some established simulation centers around the country provide workshops that provide information on starting, operating, and maintaining such a facility.[18,19] This information may be an invaluable resource for institutions and individuals who are interested in the development or improvement of their own surgical education centers.

When choosing a location for the center, it is important to keep it in as close proximity to the clinical work areas as possible (**Fig. 1**), which can sometimes be difficult to accomplish when working within an existing structure and may require creative relocation of other institutional components.[20] Even if a building outside the hospital needs to be used, easy access for faculty and trainees is paramount (**Fig. 2**). The farther the distance between the education center and the clinical workspace, the harder it is to ensure that it is used sufficiently.

Constructing a new facility to house the simulation center has the enormous advantage of allowing the building's design to concentrate mainly on the educational needs. Certain architectural firms specialize in building simulation centers but, ideally, the architects should also have expertise with the construction of medical facilities. Once again, it is essential to keep the distance between the center and the training hospital to a minimum.

Even a small center that is used only for technical skills training should provide at least 500 square feet of available simulation space.[21] It is advantageous to integrate or at least have access to a cadaver dissection laboratory and an animal OR facility, especially if there are plans to implement full procedural skills training as outlined in phase II of the National Skills Curriculum.[22] Trainees should have access to the center at all times. Many facilities, therefore, secure their education laboratory with keypad locks or require card identification for entry. The center should provide multiple workbenches, and it is critical to allow for flexible use of the available space (see **Fig. 1**). Often forgotten but of crucial importance is planning for adequate storage space.

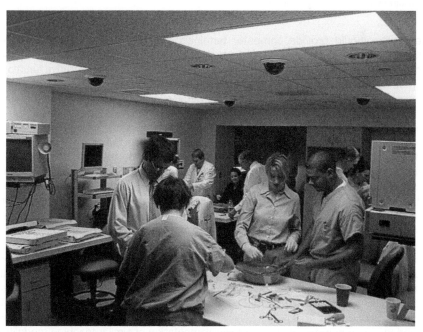

Fig. 1. The surgical skills center at the Southern Illinois University (SIU). The center contains multiple workbenches, video screens for laparoscopic skills training, and ceiling-mounted cameras to videotape the performances. The workbenches can be arranged differently to accommodate a variety of curricular activities. This space is also used for cadaver dissections. Its location across the hallway from the main OR makes it easily accessible for the residents.

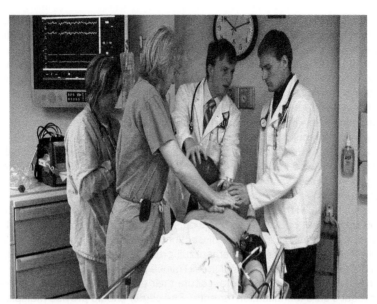

Fig. 2. The simulation center at SIU includes a patient simulation suite for patient management and team training scenarios. Because of space constraints, the suite is located in a separate location, adjacent to the sponsoring hospital. The facility is shared with other departments and is also used by the nursing staff. Its proximity to the clinical areas provides the trainees with convenient access.

The facility should provide computer terminals and Internet connections. Larger centers may want to develop a more sophisticated information technology solution, and include center-specific websites with online curricula and administrative functions such as web-based scheduling and inventory.

After allocating space for the facility, it is necessary to provide adequate staffing. First, a successful education center needs a surgical faculty member in the role of a champion who provides leadership and oversight.[21] This person is also responsible for aligning the center's activities with the curricular needs of the users. The amount of staff needed for day-to-day operations depends largely on the size and use of the facility. Even smaller centers should have at least one dedicated manager. Under ideal circumstances, the center's staff should be qualified to participate or even guide some of the educational activities. The author's center employs 1 administrative assistant and 2 surgical skills coaches with significant OR experience. The center has been able to show that these nonsurgeon skills coaches are able to teach certain basic surgical skills as effectively as an accomplished faculty educator.[23] The skills coach concept increases flexibility in providing oversight of the learners in the laboratory and decompresses the schedule of the teaching faculty. The author's center use skills coaches for a variety of its curricula, especially during the deliberate practice phase after an initial training session with a surgical faculty member. The feedback from its trainees has been overwhelmingly positive. It now seems that other education centers around the country are considering the implementation of similar teaching modalities for their programs.

Even if a center is staffed with excellent personnel, it will only flourish with a surgical faculty that accepts the concept of simulation-based training and participates in the effort. This situation is not necessarily always easy to accomplish. Especially among some more senior surgeons, the notion that surgical training should only occur in ORs, clinics, and wards remains prevalent. But even in institutions where the faculty embraces the skills laboratory as an important asset for the training program, it may remain difficult to engage them to teach within the center, as they are often already facing clinical and academic time pressure challenges that limit their availability for such activities. Support from the departmental leadership and encouragement of the faculty to participate in these teaching sessions becomes paramount for their success. Coercion may work as a method to force participation, but such a strategy most likely will not lead to a meaningful educational encounter between the faculty member and the trainees. The best way to ensure success for the education center and its curricula involves shifting the departmental culture. A surgery chairperson who elevates the importance of simulation education by making it part of the departmental value structure encourages the faculty's participation and fosters the recruitment of new faculty having genuine interest in simulation training. This approach can establish a core group of faculty members that enjoy participating in the center's educational activities and thereby improve the quality of the program. A positive faculty attitude also reflects on the trainees who realize that involvement in the center is meaningful and supported by the department and faculty. Establishing teaching awards for faculty specifically for their participation in the skills center is another mechanism of motivating them. The department at the author's center has taken this notion a step further and has developed an academic incentive program that financially rewards certain activities within the simulation center, resulting in a quarterly bonus payment.[24]

The notion "If you build it, they will come" unfortunately does not hold true for surgical education centers. Once again, it requires departmental leadership to ensure that the learners have the opportunity to use the laboratory and also to enforce their participation. Similar to faculty, trainees participate more enthusiastically when simulation and skills training represent part of the departmental educational philosophy and value system. Different models are available to integrate skills curricula with the clinical workflow and the trainee's patient service obligations, but all of them need the ongoing support of the program director and chairperson to ensure their success.

Independent practice of residents in the skills laboratory is the least disruptive method and is generally easy to implement. The curriculum can be individualized according to the learner's needs, remains flexible, and requires little faculty time. In most cases, however, this form of training will fail, because the learners often do not have the commitment to follow through. Other issues with this model are the potential lack of immediate feedback for the trainee and perceived lack of interest by the faculty to participate. Problems with oversight of the curriculum can occur as well. It is therefore better to choose a more structured approach. One possibility is to integrate the skills training into the clinical rotations. This method aligns the simulation curriculum with clinical activities and shifts the scheduling responsibility to the division responsible for the rotation. On the other hand, this approach makes it more difficult to establish a consistent curriculum of gradually increasing complexity and to confirm proficiency in certain tasks prior to allowing junior residents to perform these procedures in a clinical setting.

Some education centers have established dedicated skills rotations within their training programs.[25,26] The residents spend a certain amount of time, usually a month, within the skills laboratory and work through a defined curriculum, which provides an intense training environment and is ideal for deliberate practice. The curriculum can also be tailored to the needs of the individual. Because the activity is scheduled in advance, the trainee usually is free of any clinical service obligations. This model may not be applicable for smaller programs because of issues with service coverage. It is also important to ensure adequate oversight of the skills laboratory activity and to provide intermittent feedback to optimize the educational impact.

Another way to establish dedicated time in the education center is to schedule blocks of curricular activities, oftentimes splitting groups of residents according to their level of training. Many programs use this model for "boot camp" to prepare their new trainees for clinical activities.[27–29] The author's institution has established an intense simulation-based training program for first-year residents, which includes scheduled time in the skills laboratory 3 times a week during the first few months of their internship. The trainees follow an educational outline that is based on phase I of the National Skills Curriculum, and the faculty assesses their performance after completion of each module. The residents have no clinical obligations during this time and are required to participate. This model can have significant impact on clinical services, because multiple residents are simultaneously unavailable for ward duties at the same time. On the other hand, this training can verify the trainees' proficiency within the simulated environment before they are allowed to perform the tasks on real patients.

GOVERNANCE STRUCTURE AND FINANCIAL SUPPORT FOR THE EDUCATION CENTER

There are 2 designs for the administrative structure of a surgical education center: in one case, the center is completely managed within the surgical department; in the other, the surgical simulation program is part of a multidisciplinary center within the institution. Both models have their distinct advantages and disadvantages, and choosing one over the other depends on the given institutional environment as well as the main objectives of the center. If these objectives relate mostly to surgical skills, procedures, and patient management, and if expertise for simulation training exists within the surgical faculty, it makes sense to administer the center within the department of surgery. This structure establishes full control over the operations of the center, as well as its finances. The structure can, however, lead to substantial duplication of efforts within an institution, should other departments develop their own simulation programs. It is therefore useful to establish relationships with other institutional simulation stakeholders to coordinate efforts and share facilities and equipment where feasible in an effort to avoid this problem. In situations whereby established simulation programs already exist within an institution or if plans for the construction of a larger multidisciplinary simulation facility are under way, it may be more appropriate to integrate the surgical program into this administrative structure. Using existing expertise within the institution can be constructive in getting a new surgical program successfully off the ground and may outweigh the downside of giving up some administrative control. It remains important to identify and support a surgical faculty champion who will oversee and direct the surgical component within the center and maintain a leadership role within its administration. With the increasing interest of simulation-based training of teams, multidisciplinary approaches to simulation become more important. Logistics and implementation of such efforts may be more easily accomplished using the latter administrative model. Larger surgical programs may need to develop their own administrative infrastructure by separating operational, educational, and research components.[21]

Most surgical education centers are based within academic institutions and do not have a self-sustaining business model. It is therefore important to develop funding strategies that sustain the operations of the center. In many cases, teaching hospitals are starting to appreciate the benefits of surgical education in simulated environments, mainly with respect to quality of care and patient safety. These parameters will become increasingly important and affect hospitals' finances directly because of the ongoing changes in Medicare and the introduction of performance-based reimbursements. The willingness of teaching hospitals to provide funding for surgical education facilities will, therefore, likely continue to increase. Close collaboration with the hospital may also open additional venues for external philanthropy. Organizing tours for potential donors, holding open houses for the community, and giving presentations through local media outlets can raise public awareness for the education center and initiate new funding streams.

In the past, many education centers were at least partially funded by grants and donations from the industry. These relationships are becoming increasingly complicated because of the ongoing conflict-of-interest concerns. Many universities have implemented strict guidelines addressing collaboration with industry that have resulted in difficulties maintaining funding relationships even for purely educational purposes. It may be necessary to think creatively about the development of new funding mechanisms through the industry that are transparent, focus on educational programs, and address concerns regarding conflicts of interest between the grantor and grantee, in an effort to continue these important relationships in the future.

Another avenue of financial support of these facilities is through competitive research grants. This mechanism may be more appropriate for larger centers with an established research agenda, because most of these grants are becoming significantly more competitive.

A few education centers have been successful in funding a portion of the educational enterprise through continuing medical education (CME) courses or by opening their facility for educational activities provided by industry, usually to introduce new technologies to surgeons in practice. CME activities often require substantial resources and may therefore not provide as much revenue as anticipated. Collaboration with industry can be very successful as a funding model but, as mentioned earlier, these relationships need to be scrutinized in the academic setting to avoid conflicts of interest.

DEVELOPMENT AND STRUCTURING OF THE CURRICULUM FOR THE EDUCATION CENTER

One major advantage of moving the educational platform from the clinical to a simulated environment is the increased ability to plan the curriculum. Traditional training depended mostly on random patient flow through the clinical services,[30] resulting in learning by "random opportunity." Surgical education laboratories allow us to organize the curriculum in a stepwise fashion according to the learner needs and level of training. Moreover, simulation allows the learner to fail safely in a supportive environment and to learn from such experiences, whereas failure in the clinical setting caused by inexperience is truly no longer a feasible option. A variety of studies have shown that simulation training can move the learning curve outside of the OR, thereby potentially decreasing OR time.[31,32] In another study, after a month of following the simulation curriculum, students reached a level of expertise similar to that of a resident in performing basic surgical skills.[33] The training occurs in a structured and repeatable fashion and provides opportunity for directed feedback, making training in the skills laboratory an ideal place for deliberate practice, which, according to Ericsson,[34] is a crucial component in developing expertise. Surgical education centers are also well suited to address the issue of the "July phenomenon," or the entrance of neophyte trainees into the clinical workplace.[35] Simulation curricula have been implemented successfully during the fourth year of medical school and just before the beginning of clinical rotations in an effort to prepare the new residents for their clinical duties.[36,37] Ideally, educational simulation activities should be aligned with already existing clinical curricula, if feasible,[38] to strengthen their educational impact. The education center can also be used to improve strategies for recognition and remedi-ation of the marginal resident because currently, significant delays in identification and intervention for these individuals seem to be a frequent problem.[39]

Surgeons tend to conceptually reduce simulation to mere technical skills training using models, box trainers, and VR devices. Such an attitude may unnecessarily narrow the curricular activities within the education center. Simulation is capable of covering a much broader training agenda. Even in the surgical field, additional educa-tional modalities such as standardized patients integrate well into the curriculum. Kneebone's work at Imperial College in London has demonstrated well how a combi-nation of the task trainer and simulated patient can provide an additional dimension and incorporate the task performance into a clinical context.[40–42] The program at the author's center has included standardized outpatient clinic scenarios and patient assessment and management examinations[43] for many years to assess residents during patient encounters and to provide them with directed feedback on their performance.

The success of surgical education centers depends mainly on the quality of the curriculum. Educational activities need to be well thought out, a process that is much more important than simulation technology itself.[21] Many programs have failed because they used available funding to purchase simulation equipment and only then tried to figure out what to use it for. It cannot be overemphasized that curriculum development needs to come first and also follow sound educational principles. The process can be fairly labor intensive and usually includes a formal assessment of needs of the learners, followed by the definition of learning goals and objectives. The curriculum is then designed and implemented. It is important to obtain feedback from the learners and educators and to adjust the curriculum based on this feedback. Decisions regarding equipment needs should be based solely on the learning objec-tives that were obtained from this process. In many situations, these objectives can be met using low-fidelity equipment. Many skills sessions in the author's center make extensive use of self-made, low-cost, reusable models and still accomplish the required learning goals (**Fig. 3**).

Developing new curricula is not easy, especially for small programs that are just beginning to use simulation as part of their training program. In an effort to facilitate this process, the American College of Surgeons (ACS)/Association of Program Direc-tors in Surgery (APDS) National Surgical Skills Curriculum was developed.[22] The curriculum is available online (http://elearning.facs.org) and contains a large body of skills and procedural modules, team training exercises, assessment tools, and other associated content. These materials can be used free of charge.

The enormous progress in computer processing speed and imaging capabilities has led to dramatic developments in the area of surgical simulation. VR simulation soft-ware that required workstations costing $150,000 10 years ago can now be imple-mented on high-end laptops. The ability to simulate haptics, thereby allowing the user to "feel" the virtual environment, has also markedly improved. At present, a large variety of VR simulators are commercially available, many of them offering built-in curricula, automated testing, and tools to assess performance.[44] Despite such impressive capabilities, the debate regarding any added educational benefit of VR over less realistic but substantially cheaper simulators continues. It also remains to be seen whether the additional expense for haptic capability provides any significant

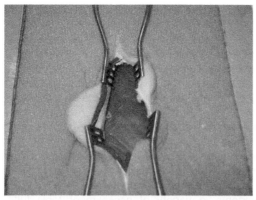

Fig. 3. Example of a low-cost, self-made model for surgical skills. This model can be used to practice the laparotomy incision and fascial closure as outlined in module 12 in phase I of the National Surgical Skills Curriculum. It takes approximately 15 minutes to make it and costs $8. Detailed instructions on how to create the model are available online. (*Data from* Ketchum J, Bartlett J. Southern Illinois School of Medicine laparotomy model. Available at: http://elearning.facs.org/mod/resource/view.php?id=449. Updated 2009. Accessed October 29, 2009.)

advantage.[45,46] One of the best studied and validated laparoscopic skills curricula to date is the Fundamentals of Laparoscopic Surgery skills program,[47–50] which uses a simple videoscopic box trainer. Multiple studies have demonstrated transfer of skill for laparoscopic procedures using low- and high-fidelity simulators,[13,17] but the superiority of VR simulation over simple box trainers has not been established.[51] Many of the VR simulators store a large amount of data regarding a user's performance, but only some of these data correlate well with clinical assessment.[52] A recent study suggests that measuring task completion time alone may provide the best measurement to assess task proficiency.[53] At this point, it is not possible to make definitive statements regarding the utility of low- versus high-fidelity surgical simulators, especially as the realism of the VR environments continues to improve. High-fidelity simulators provide an exciting area for ongoing research, and they may open up new venues to optimize procedural training for surgical residents.[54] These simulators can also be used as an effective public relations tool during promotional events for the surgical education center. The recent development of rehearsal simulations in interventional carotid stenting using patient-specific data sets demonstrates the enormous potential of this technology in the future.[55,56]

As mentioned earlier, decisions regarding the purchase of surgical simulators should be based mostly on the curricular learning objectives. The best philosophy regarding the education center is not to view it as purely a showroom for new simulation technology but as a functional extension and improvement of the educational mission within the department and institution.

ASSESSING PERFORMANCE, PROGRESS, AND COMPETENCY

The ACGME outcomes project, which was launched in 1999, resulted in an increased focus on assessment of performance and competence for medical students and residents. The surgical skills center provides an ideal setting to perform these assessments in a safe and reproducible environment. It is also evident from the literature that assessment and formative feedback serve a valid educational purpose,[57] especially when provided shortly after the performance. All curricular activities should therefore include an assessment of the learner. Nevertheless, formal assessment of resident performance in the surgical skills laboratory is currently not widely implemented and is mostly performed at institutions having an established track record in surgical education research. This situation may be caused by increasing time constraints on surgical faculty and the lack of structural integration of such assessments into the overall evaluation process of the residents in most institutions. Many residency programs may feel overwhelmed and lack sufficient expertise to develop such assessment instruments themselves. In an effort to promote assessment in surgical skills centers across the country, it is important to provide assessment instruments that are easy to access and use, and that provide valid results. With the development of the ACS/APDS Surgical Skills Curriculum for residents, a variety of assessment tools fulfilling these criteria have become available.[58] The assessment process can be streamlined further using modern video capture technology. For the last year, the author's institution has used such technology to assess postgraduate year 1 residents. The trainees' performance is captured on video and distributed online to the assessing faculty member. The reviewers can access the video from their office through a standard Web browser. The assessment instrument appears automatically when reviewing the video and is completed online (**Fig. 4**). All assessment forms are stored centrally on the server and remain available for reporting purposes. The reviewing faculty member can also annotate segments of the video, thereby providing directed feedback for the trainee.

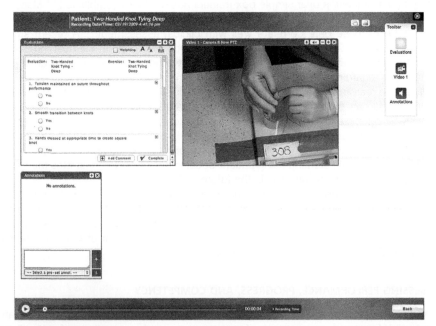

Fig. 4. Web-based skills assessment tool. The reviewer has online access to the video of the performance, the task-specific assessment instrument, and an annotation window to give directed feedback to the trainee.

ACS EDUCATION INSTITUTE ACCREDITATION PROCESS

The ACS Education Institute program was created in an effort to enhance patient safety, address the core competencies for residents and surgeons, and enable access to contemporary surgical education through the support of simulation-based surgical education.[59] The program also provides a network of institutions to encourage the exchange of expertise and to foster collaborative education research. At present, almost 50 surgical education centers have been accredited, including centers in England, Sweden, and Greece. Accreditation is offered at 2 levels and involves a vigorous assessment of the institute's cohort of learners, curricula, and available resources. The application process is fairly labor intensive, but it enables the applying center to formally analyze its current activities, strengths, and weaknesses and to develop strategic plans for the future.[60] The evaluation focuses heavily on sound educational principles, curriculum development, and educational research, especially for the comprehensive level I centers, and provides a seal of approval for the successful institutions.[61] The ACS was the first national organization to develop such a formalized process. Since then, other organizations have begun their own accreditation processes.

SUMMARY

Surgical education centers can add tremendous value to the education program of a surgical department. Their success, however, depends largely on the strong support by the leadership of the department and residency program, and on the identification of a faculty member for the role of the center's champion. It is important to clearly identify the center's goals and objectives, and to choose a suitable structure for governance. The center's curricula should be integrated into the residency training program, and infrastructure that ensures faculty participation should be developed. Sound educational methodology should be implemented, and the center's focus should be directed toward curricular development before considering the purchase of simulator equipment. Following these principles should make the surgical education center successful, whether it is small or large.

REFERENCES

1. Mayberry JC. Residency reform Halsted-style. J Am Coll Surg 2003;197(3): 433–5.
2. Rogers RG. Teaching and evaluating surgical skills. Obstet Gynecol Clin North Am 2006;33(2):xv–xvi.
3. Kohn L, Corrigan J, Donaldson M. To err is human. Washington, DC: National Academies Press; 1999.
4. Weatherby BA, Rudd JN, Ervin TB, et al. The effect of resident work hour regulations on orthopaedic surgical education. J Surg Orthop Adv 2007;16(1):19–22.
5. Whang EE, Perez A, Ito H, et al. Work hours reform: perceptions and desires of contemporary surgical residents. J Am Coll Surg 2003;197(4):624–30.
6. Bridges M, Diamond DL. The financial impact of teaching surgical residents in the operating room. Am J Surg 1999;177(1):28–32.
7. Harrington DT, Roye GD, Ryder BA, et al. A time-cost analysis of teaching a laparoscopic entero-enterostomy. J Surg Educ 2007;64(6):342–5.
8. Gaba DM. Improving anesthesiologists' performance by simulating reality. Anesthesiology 1992;76(4):491–4.

9. Gaba DM, DeAnda A. A comprehensive anesthesia simulation environment: recreating the operating room for research and training. Anesthesiology 1988; 69(3):387–94.

10. ACGME. The ACGME outcomes project. Available at: http://www.acgme.org/outcome/. Accessed October 23, 2009.

11. Dunnington GL, Williams RG. Addressing the new competencies for residents' surgical training. Acad Med 2003;78(1):14–21.

12. Torkington J, Smith SG, Rees BI, et al. Skill transfer from virtual reality to a real laparoscopic task. Surg Endosc 2001;15(10):1076–9.

13. Seymour NE, Gallagher AG, Roman SA, et al. Virtual reality training improves operating room performance: results of a randomized, double-blinded study. Ann Surg 2002;236(4):458–63 [discussion: 463–4].

14. Residency Review Committee for General Surgery. ACGME program requirements for graduate medical education in surgery. Available at: http://www.acgme.org/acWebsite/downloads/RRC_progReq/440_general_surgery_01012008_u08102008.pdf; 2008. Accessed October 1, 2009.

15. Gould JC. Building a laparoscopic surgical skills training laboratory: resources and support. JSLS 2006;10(3):293–6.

16. Acker L. Overcoming operational challenges: an administrator's perspective. In: Kyle R, Murray W, editors. Clinical simulation—operations, engineering, and management. Boston: Elsevier; 2008. p. 59–67.

17. Aggarwal R, Ward J, Balasundaram I, et al. Proving the effectiveness of virtual reality simulation for training in laparoscopic surgery. Ann Surg 2007;246(5): 771–9.

18. Sanfey H, Dunnington G, Ketchum J, et al. Surgical skills lab workshops. Available at: http://www.siumed.edu/surgery/surgical_skills/surgical_skills_workshop.html. Accessed October 27, 2009.

19. Dunn W, Coltvet G, Belda T, et al. From the ground up: simulation center building blocks—creating a simulation center. Available at: http://www.mayo.edu/simulationcenter/Designing-A-Center-Course.html. Accessed October 27, 2009.

20. Wiley E, Murray W. Educational needs dictating learning space: factors considered in the identification and planning of appropriate space for a simulation learning complex. In: Kyle R, Murray W, editors. Clinical simulation—operations, engineering, and management. Boston: Elsevier; 2008. p. 301–17.

21. Qayumi K. Centers of excellence: a new dimension in surgical education. Surg Innov 2006;13(2):120–8.

22. Scott DJ, Dunnington GL. The new ACS/APDS skills curriculum: moving the learning curve out of the operating room. J Gastrointest Surg 2008;12(2): 213–21.

23. Kim M, Boehler M, Ketchum J, et al. Skills coaches as part of the educational team: a randomized controlled trial of teaching of a basic surgical skill in the laboratory setting. Am J Surg 2010;199(1):94–8.

24. Williams RG, Dunnington GL, Folse JR. The impact of a program for systematically recognizing and rewarding academic performance. Acad Med 2003; 78(2):156–66.

25. Foley PJ, Dumon KR, Roses RE, et al. A dedicated one-month laparoscopic and endoscopic skills rotation significantly improves surgical residents' technical skill and reduces error scores. J Am Coll Surg 2008;207(3 Suppl 1):S94.

26. Gonzalez RI, Martinez JM, Iglesias AR, et al. Technical skills rotation for general surgery residents. J Surg Res 2009;151(2):285.

27. Esterl RM Jr, Henzi DL, Cohn SM. Senior medical student "Boot Camp": can result in increased self-confidence before starting surgery internships. Curr Surg 2006; 63(4):264–8.
28. Fann JI, Calhoon JH, Carpenter AJ, et al. Simulation in coronary artery anastomosis early in cardiothoracic surgical residency training: the Boot Camp experience. J Thorac Cardiovasc Surg, in press.
29. Vergara VM, Panaiotis, Kingsley D, et al. The use of virtual reality simulation of head trauma in a surgical boot camp. Stud Health Technol Inform 2009;142:395–7.
30. Gorman PJ, Meier AH, Rawn C, et al. The future of medical education is no longer blood and guts, it is bits and bytes. Am J Surg 2000;180(5):353–6.
31. Larsen CR, Soerensen JL, Grantcharov TP, et al. Effect of virtual reality training on laparoscopic surgery: randomised controlled trial. BMJ 2009;338:b1802.
32. Sturm LP, Windsor JA, Cosman PH, et al. A systematic review of skills transfer after surgical simulation training. Ann Surg 2008;248(2):166–79.
33. Boehler ML, Schwind CJ, Rogers DA, et al. A theory-based curriculum for enhancing surgical skillfulness. J Am Coll Surg 2007;205(3):492–7.
34. Ericsson KA. Deliberate practice and the acquisition and maintenance of expert performance in medicine and related domains. Acad Med 2004;79(Suppl 10): S70–81.
35. Dutta S, Dunnington G, Blanchard MC, et al. And doctor, no residents please!. J Am Coll Surg 2003;197(6):1012–7.
36. Boehler ML, Rogers DA, Schwind CJ, et al. A senior elective designed to prepare medical students for surgical residency. Am J Surg 2004;187(6):695–7.
37. Meier AH, Henry J, Marine R, et al. Implementation of a web- and simulation-based curriculum to ease the transition from medical school to surgical internship. Am J Surg 2005;190(1):137–40.
38. Beeman L. Integration of simulation with existing clinical education programs. In: Kyle R, Murray W, editors. Clinical simulation—operations, engineering, and management. Boston: Elsevier; 2008. p. 109–26.
39. Williams RG, Roberts NK, Schwind CJ, et al. The nature of general surgery resident performance problems. Surgery 2009;145(6):651–8.
40. Black SA, Nestel DF, Horrocks EJ, et al. Evaluation of a framework for case development and simulated patient training for complex procedures. Simul Healthc 2006;1(2):66–71.
41. Kneebone R, Nestel D, Yadollahi F, et al. Assessing procedural skills in context: exploring the feasibility of an integrated procedural performance instrument (IPPI). Med Educ 2006;40(11):1105–14.
42. Kneebone RL, Nestel D, Moorthy K, et al. Learning the skills of flexible sigmoidoscopy—the wider perspective. Med Educ 2003;37(Suppl 1):50–8.
43. MacRae H, Regehr G, Leadbetter W, et al. A comprehensive examination for senior surgical residents. Am J Surg 2000;179(3):190–3.
44. Scott DJ, Cendan JC, Pugh CM, et al. The changing face of surgical education: simulation as the new paradigm. J Surg Res 2008;147(2):189–93.
45. Panait L, Akkary E, Bell RL, et al. The role of haptic feedback in laparoscopic simulation training. J Surg Res 2009;156(2):312–6.
46. Shamsunder SC, Manivannan M. Haptic guided laparoscopy simulation improves learning curve. Stud Health Technol Inform 2008;132:454–6.
47. Feldman LS, Cao J, Andalib A, et al. A method to characterize the learning curve for performance of a fundamental laparoscopic simulator task: defining "learning plateau" and "learning rate". Surgery 2009;146(2):381–6.

48. Scott DJ, Ritter EM, Tesfay ST, et al. Certification pass rate of 100% for fundamentals of laparoscopic surgery skills after proficiency-based training. Surg Endosc 2008;22(8):1887–93.
49. Fried GM. FLS assessment of competency using simulated laparoscopic tasks. J Gastrointest Surg 2008;12(2):210–2.
50. McCluney AL, Vassiliou MC, Kaneva PA, et al. FLS simulator performance predicts intraoperative laparoscopic skill. Surg Endosc 2007;21(11):1991–5.
51. Botden SM, Torab F, Buzink SN, et al. The importance of haptic feedback in laparoscopic suturing training and the additive value of virtual reality simulation. Surg Endosc 2008;22(5):1214–22.
52. Wohaibi EM, Bush RW, Earle DB, et al. Surgical resident performance on a virtual reality simulator correlates with operating room performance. J Surg Res, in press.
53. Stefanidis D, Scott DJ, Korndorffer JR Jr. Do metrics matter? Time versus motion tracking for performance assessment of proficiency-based laparoscopic skills training. Simul Healthc 2009;4(2):104–8.
54. Kishore TA, Beddingfield R, Holden T, et al. Task deconstruction facilitates acquisition of transurethral resection of prostate skills on a virtual reality trainer. J Endourol 2009;23(4):665–8.
55. Roguin A, Beyar R. Real case virtual reality training prior to carotid artery stenting. Catheter Cardiovasc Interv, in press.
56. Hislop SJ, Hedrick JH, Singh MJ, et al. Simulation case rehearsals for carotid artery stenting. Eur J Vasc Endovasc Surg, in press.
57. Boehler ML, Rogers DA, Schwind CJ, et al. An investigation of medical student reactions to feedback: a randomised controlled trial. Med Educ 2006;40(8): 746–9.
58. ACS/APDS. Verification of proficiency modules. Available at: http://elearning. facs.org/mod/resource/view.php?id=281. Accessed October 24, 2009.
59. Sachdeva AK, Pellegrini CA, Johnson KA. Support for simulation-based surgical education through American College of Surgeons-accredited education institutes. World J Surg 2008;32(2):196–207.
60. Johnson KA, Sachdeva AK, Pellegrini CA. The critical role of accreditation in establishing the ACS Education Institutes to advance patient safety through simulation. J Gastrointest Surg 2008;12(2):207–9.
61. ACS. Program requirements. Available at: http://www.facs.org/education/ accreditationprogram/requirements.html. Accessed October 10, 2009.

Focused Surgical Skills Training for Senior Medical Students and Interns

Mary E. Klingensmith, MD*, L. Michael Brunt, MD

KEYWORDS

- Simulation • Surgical education
- Undergraduate medical education
- Graduate medical education • Surgical residency training

Surgical skills laboratories have become an increasingly important component of technical skills training for learners entering surgical fields. The advantages of learning in the skills laboratory are that they provide an opportunity to learn in a low-stress environment, free from ethical concerns of patient safety. Rare events can also be practiced in the skills laboratory arena, making trainees more capable of handling the technical demands necessary, should such an event be encountered in surgical practice (ie, need for an emergent surgical airway). With regard to learners entering surgical fields, skills laboratories can provide motivation and direction for students and residents, directing their practice to relevant areas.[1] Indeed, the Accreditation Council for Graduate Medical Education (ACGME) has acknowledged the value of skills laboratories, making them a mandatory part of surgical residency training for maintenance of program accreditation as of July 2008.

Intensive skills training for senior medical students who are planning careers in surgery have become increasingly common.[2,3] Typically held in the spring of the senior year, these courses intend to provide intensive task training in techniques and skills that these learners will need for proficient performance as a surgical intern. The value of these courses and the need to consider standardization across medical schools culminated in the formation, in 2009, of a committee by the American College of Surgeons (ACS), the Association for Surgical Education, and the Association of Program Directors in Surgery (APDS) to examine these issues.

In this article the authors summarize their current experience with intern and senior medical student curricula, as well as that of others. Advantages and limitations of this approach to training are explored.

Department of Surgery, Washington University School of Medicine, Campus PO Box 8109, 660 South Euclid, Saint Louis, MO 63110, USA
* Corresponding author.
E-mail address: klingensmithm@wustl.edu

Surg Clin N Am 90 (2010) 505–518
doi:10.1016/j.suc.2010.02.004
0039-6109/10/$ – see front matter. Published by Elsevier Inc.

surgical.theclinics.com

SKILLS PREPARATION FOR SENIOR MEDICAL STUDENTS

Medical students may lag in skills development for many of the same reasons that impinge on surgical interns and junior residents. The clinical rotations of medical students vary widely, and many spend only 4 weeks on a core surgical rotation in the third year. Surgical subinternship experience in the fourth year is also highly variable. The pressures for increased operating room (OR) efficiency may further limit students' hands-on skills development in the OR. The work hour restrictions for medical students and the reduced night-call frequency may negatively impact their preparedness for internship as well.

Despite the widespread recognition of the importance of skills training in surgical residency, in recent years only a few institutions have reported the implementation of skills training courses that target the preparedness of senior medical students for surgical internship.[2–4] These courses have taken a variety of formats and have incorporated didactic and hands-on training. The format of such courses has varied from a 1-month long elective period to more broadly spaced sessions that are given periodically over several weeks.

In 2006, in an effort to begin to address some of these concerns as well as our perceived anecdotal observation of deficient baseline intern skills sets, we (the authors of this article) established a skills course in the spring of the senior year for senior students who were matching in a surgical specialty, which we called "Accelerated Skills Preparation for Surgical Internship." The course entails 7 3-hour sessions given weekly, baseline pre- and postcourse skills assessment, and a final written examination. The basic structure of each session consisted of a short lecture followed by hands-on skills training and practice. Each session was led by an attending surgeon with assistance from surgical residents, most of whom had completed 2 or 3 years of clinical training. A brief description of the course is given in the following sections.

Session 1: Basic Suturing and Knot Tying and Surgical Instruments

Surgical instruments are reviewed, and an overview of the basics of suture materials, suturing, and knot-tying principles is presented. Students then practice these skills in small groups led by a resident instructor. Students are given suturing instruments, a knot-tying board, and a suturing pad to keep until the end of the rotation, and are expected to practice regularly. In addition, a comprehensive set of videos demonstrating suturing and tying is made available for Web-based viewing.

Session 2: Common Management Problems on the Patient Floor

The initial assessment and management of the patient with chest pain, shortness of breath, hypotension, fever, arrhythmia, respiratory and cardiac arrest, and other postoperative and acute on-call problems is reviewed. Case scenarios are presented and discussed in small breakout groups, with an emphasis on communication skills.

Session 3: Emergent Procedural Techniques

The basics of intubation, central-line placement, chest tube insertion, surgical airway, intravenous (IV)-line placement, and arterial puncture are reviewed. These skills are then practiced using various models and manikins.

Session 4: Use of Surgical Staplers and Surgical Energy Devices

The principles and basic techniques for the use of electrocautery, ultrasonic energy devices, and mechanical staplers are reviewed. Students practice with these devices on various ex vivo models, perform a simulated excisional biopsy, and are instructed on the use of local anesthetic technique.

Session 5: Basic Laparoscopic Skills and Drills

The basics of laparoscopic instrumentation and video imaging systems are reviewed; students learn and practice basic laparoscopic skills and camera navigation in a trainer box using the Society of American Gastrointestinal and Endoscopic Surgeons' Fundamentals of Laparoscopic Surgery (FLS) program. A simulated laparoscopic cholecystectomy is also performed using an explanted porcine liver. An FLS instructional video is given to each student and they are provided with access to a laparoscopic trainer box for further practice.

Session 6: Trauma Evaluation and Management: Adaptation of Advanced Trauma Life Support

The Trauma Evaluation and Management program derived from the ACS' Advanced Trauma Life Support course is reviewed. Students are oriented to the initial evaluation and early management of the patient with trauma, and are instructed on how to care for patients with life-threatening or potentially life-threatening injuries.

Session 7: Animate Skills Laboratory

This final instructional session consists of a 6-hour laboratory work in which the students have the opportunity to apply the skills that they have learned in the previous sessions on a live porcine model. Procedures covered include laparoscopic access and laparoscopic cholecystectomy, opening and closing the abdomen, intestinal resection and anastomosis, solid organ resection, chest tube insertion, and surgical airway. Students perform a hand-sutured and mechanical-stapled intestinal anastomosis. The essentials of being a good surgical assistant are also emphasized.

Session 8: Assessment

Students are given a written examination covering the practical knowledge and skills acquired during the previous sessions. In addition, postcourse testing of suturing and knot-tying skills is performed.

Other Curricular Options

Additional topics that have been incorporated into senior skills curricula at other institutions include sessions such as anatomy instruction with cadaver dissection, standardized patient experiences, mock pages, and intensive care unit rounds. The senior skills course at Southern Illinois University (SIU) includes several mock page scenarios in which students respond to pages about hypothetical patients and are then given immediate feedback.[2] We found that students' anxiety level about starting internship was highest for managing acute on-call problems. Another approach to address this shortcoming would be to develop standardized emergency room and/or night-call rotations that give students the experience in dealing with acute emergencies and on-call problems to which they get little exposure today and yet, as interns, are asked to deal with regularly when on call.

Results of Assessment

Assessment of performance and knowledge acquisition has been an important component of our senior skills course in order to measure the impact of the skills being taught and to drive and motivate learning. The results of assessment data from the first 2 years of the course in which 31 students were enrolled were recently reported.[3] We tested performance on 5 basic suturing and knot-tying tasks, namely, simple interrupted suturing, subcuticular closure, 1- and 2-handed knot tying, and knot tying in a restricted space with an instrument pass. Task times improved significantly post course for all tasks except 2-handed knot tying. Before the course, the total time required to complete all 5 tasks was 848 ± 214 seconds compared with 677 ± 151 seconds post course ($P<.0001$), representing an average reduction in total task time of almost 3 minutes. We also compared the performance of students on these tasks with that of end of second year general surgery residents. Post course, the residents were significantly faster for only 1-handed knot tying and tying in a restricted space, but not for the other tasks. On postcourse laparoscopic skills testing, 11 of 19 students were able to pass all 5 components of the FLS skills examination.[5] Finally, more than 80% of students achieved a proficiency score in the final written examination (LM Brunt, unpublished data, 2009).

Self-assessment of confidence levels regarding their preparedness for internship was performed for 45 domains related to management of acute patient care problems and basic procedural and technical skills using a 1- to 5-point Likert scale (1 = no knowledge, unable to perform up to 5 = highly knowledgable, confident, and independent).[3] Mean student self-assessment scores for all 45 questions combined increased significantly from 3.2 ± 1.3 pre-course to 3.9 ± 0.6 post course. Students indicated that their knowledge and confidence levels were low (mean score ≤2.5) pre-course for 13 of 45 questions (28.8%), compared with the knowledge and confidence levels (mean score ≤2.5) post course for none of the questions. Reasonably confident or highly knowledgable and confident/independent mean scores (≥4.0) were seen for only 26.7% of questions pre-course compared with 48.9% of questions post course.

Similar findings regarding an increased sense of preparedness have been reported by other groups. Peyre and colleagues[6] found that confidence levels of 6 senior medical students who undertook a skills preparation course not only improved significantly but also was higher than the confidence levels of incoming interns. Esterl and colleagues[7] showed a similar degree of improvement in confidence levels across 4 broad areas after a 4-week senior "boot camp" skills elective. In another study, introduction of a simulation and Web-based curriculum for managing on-call problems during intern orientation improved confidence levels for managing these types of problems.[8] In terms of knowledge acquisition, Boehler and colleagues[2] found that post-course examination scores were not only higher than pre-course scores but also were significantly higher than those of surgical interns. Despite these results, further studies are needed to determine if improved performance in the skills laboratory and increased confidence levels translate into actual improved performance in the OR or in clinical rotations.

Resources

A major challenge to putting on skills courses for senior medical students is the time and expense involved. Because all programs now have mandated skills laboratories for residency training, the course content and other resources should be complementary with those used for resident training. Substantial time and effort was initially invested in developing the structure and didactic content of the various sessions in our course, but this material is now becoming standardized and can be taken from existing courses or from the National Skills Curriculum. Support personnel (ie, an education coordinator), who can assist with planning of sessions and ensuring that the appropriate supplies and resources are made available, is essential. Our institution has a part-time surgical education coordinator and a fulltime registered nurse education coordinator at the Simulation Center in the School of Medicine. These coordinators have been invaluable in performing the operational aspects of the course. Each session is staffed with a faculty instructor as well as resident laboratory instructors, who can provide individual and small group instructions and feedback for the various skills.

Funding for the course initially came from a pilot grant from Washington University, and has been further supported by educational grants and in-kind support from industry. Some up-front capital equipment purchases that included central and IV-line manikins, laparoscopic surgery trainer boxes, and surgical instrument sets for suturing practice were made for our course. A list of essential equipment for our fourth year course is listed in **Box 1**. Current annual capital cost per student for the course is approximately $300. Education coordinator's support time for planning and execution

---

Box 1
Sample equipment list for senior medical student skills course

Suturing and knot-tying materials

    Silicone suture pads

    Knot-tying boards

    Instrument set (needle driver, Debakey and Adson forceps, scissors)

    Suture material

    Surgical instrument tray

Emergent surgical procedures

    Intubation: manikin (adult and pediatric)

    Central-line simulation manikin with placement torso

    Central-line kit

    Chest-tube insertion: chest tubes, rib specimens, IV bag

    IV line: IV arm manikin, 20-gauge IV catheters, IV tubing and fluids, alcohol swabs, IV dressing

Laparoscopic skills

    Laparoscopic tower with basic laparoscopic equipment and instrumentation (graspers, scissors, hook cautery, and other instruments)

    Trainer box with FLS-skills drills and pretied loop sutures

    Camera navigation setup

    Explanted porcine liver for laparoscopic cholecystectomy

Energy sources and surgical stapling devices

    Electrocautery unit with pencil tip cautery

    Ultrasonic and/or bipolar coagulating devices

    Linear cutter and thoracoabdominal (TA) type staplers with multiple reloads

    Foam for stapler applications

    Chicken pieces for cautery and energy device practice

    Grapes, olives, or similar for implant excision

    10-mL syringes and 22- or 25-gauge needles

    Forceps, curved dissecting clamp

of the course, including class time, has ranged from 50 to 60 hours. Additional staff time may be needed for assessment and will vary, depending on what skills are tested and whether testing is done baseline as well as post course.

INTERN SKILLS TRAINING
Washington University Experience

Since 2001, the first author (M.E.K.) has overseen an intensive summer session of skills laboratories for interns. Over time, the offering has expanded to its current structure (**Box 2**). Sessions are held weekly for 2 hours, during which time the interns are relieved of all clinical duties. All sessions are held during the summer months, with the goal of covering all content early in the training experience. From the outset, our curriculum has been formative, intending to ensure that all trainees have basic instruction in techniques, which we believe is important for all our junior residents to possess. In some cases, these sessions introduce interns to procedures for the first time (ie, cricothyroidotomy), and in other cases they reinforce and build on nascent skills (ie, knot tying). Early in our experience we performed a needs assessment of our learners and discovered widely disparate experiences with these basic skills and knowledge sets.[9] The current curriculum has evolved based on intern and senior resident input as well as on faculty direction regarding gaps in skills and knowledge. Unlike other programs,[10] we have traditionally had no assessment or summative component to our program, instead intending for the curriculum to be instructive and to provide motivation and direction for further practice by trainees. However, in the 2009 to 2010 academic year we began a program that included an initial evaluation of suturing and knot-tying skills, intensive guided practice, and a follow-up assessment of these skills after 3 months. The goal of this assessment is to provide further motivation and direction for practice, and to identify those individuals in need of remedial training.

The residency program at Washington University typically has 25 interns each year. Our sessions are held in a variety of locations around our campus, depending on the topic, ranging from a task training room in our Simulation Center (**Fig. 1**) to our minimally invasive training laboratory (**Fig. 2**). Learner to instructor ratio is kept in the 3:1 to 6:1 range. Instructors include chief residents, fellows, and faculty members, although we have included industry representatives on occasion, especially for the stapling and energy source sessions (see **Box 2**). As detailed in **Box 2**, most sessions are task-training oriented, typically using low-tech devices and instruments. Cast-off instruments and outdated supplies from our hospital's ORs have been a rich source for much of our needed equipment and supplies. We are fortunate to have a large training program in graduate medical education (GME) at our medical center and have been able to leverage this into shared resources for some of our sessions (ie, CVC insertion and airway management). Nevertheless, sessions involving cadavers or live porcine models are expensive. Further, the time that faculty contribute to teaching in these sessions is also valuable, because the traditional means of teaching (in the OR or at the bedside) are part of the typical revenue stream for a surgeon. These sessions are completely out of that revenue stream and as such, the motivations to teach can be difficult to achieve. We do not specifically remunerate our faculty who teach in these sessions, although there are faculty incentive structures for this, as described elsewhere.[11]

Throughout the remainder of the academic year, we have a variety of instructional sessions in our skills and simulation laboratories for trainees of all levels. Interns specifically will gain additional experience in topics such as handsewn vascular and intestinal anastomosis, endoscopy and laparoscopy using high-fidelity simulators, inguinal hernia repair, axillary dissection, and introduction to team training. Each of these sessions tends to be directed to our categorical trainees.

CVC insertion training at Washington University

With regard to CVC training for all interns, we have been fortunate to have considerable shared resources at our disposal for intensive training.[12] In 2006, our hospital formed an initiative aimed at improving patient safety related to CVC insertion. A committee was formed comprising members from the Departments of Medicine, Surgery, Radiology, Emergency Medicine, Anesthesiology, Neurology, and Obstetrics and Gynecology, with an intent to develop a common training program for CVC insertion and to address several components of patient safety inherent in this common bedside procedure. Surveys and case log data were used to assess previous experience with CVC placement among our trainees. Our team then used Failure Mode and Effects Analysis (FMEA) to identify high-priority failure modes, which informed the development of a curriculum that contains standard content as well as items that are specifically designed to address 3 high-profile targets.

The current curriculum content facilitates acquisition of the skills, knowledge, and behaviors that are needed to decrease the frequency, diminish the severity, and improve the early detection of the failure modes identified in our analysis. In our curriculum, training on maximum sterile barriers was designed to address catheter-related bloodstream infections; training on catheter and guidewire techniques was developed to avoid retained guidewires; and training for ultrasound-guided vascular access was designed to address arterial punctures. The curriculum is delivered as didactic content in an online format, as well as in hands-on training modules. Trainees are required to complete these online modules during and before intern orientation at the start of the academic year. Groups of trainees then come to the Simulation Center for a multistation hands-on training session that incorporates elements intended to teach the psychomotor components of the CVC insertion task (ie, proper Seldinger technique) as well as the judgment required for safe insertion (ie, common sources of error, interpretation of chest radiographs, and use of checklists). Trainee progress is tracked using multiple assessments, including multiple-choice quizzes and checklist-guided assessment of CVC insertion in a simulated environment; these assessments are done prior to the start of internship and again later in the academic year after a minimum of 5 proctored insertions have been placed in the clinical setting. Through our experience we have recognized that FMEA can provide a process for converting data from multiple sources into learning objectives, and we are investigating this technique as a means to inform curriculum development for other skills curricula.

ACS/APDS Skills Curriculum

In anticipation of skills laboratories being incorporated into the accreditation requirements for residency programs in July 2008, a committee led by Drs Gary Dunnington, Debra DaRosa, and Helen McRae was formed in 2005 by a combined effort of ACS and APDS.[10] The objective of the committee was to improve resident performance through skills-laboratory practice and to improve determination of OR readiness through standardized assessment.[10] The ACS/APDS National Skills Curriculum that resulted out of this committee's work includes 3 phases. Phase I is most relevant to the focused teaching of senior medical students and interns; this phase includes basic technical skills common to junior surgical trainees, for the most part, regardless of future intended surgical subspecialization. The modules included in phase I are listed in **Box 3**. This curriculum is available to all trainees free of charge. Included in each module are explicit instructions for skills-laboratory coordinators and instructors,

Box 2
Current Washington University "intern boot camp" schedule

Instrument basics

    Identifying common instruments

    Basics of instrument use

    Use of laparotomy instrument pan from OR

Suturing basics

    1- and 2-handed knot tying

    Subcuticular, simple interrupted, vertical, and horizontal mattress suturing

    Use of knot-tying boards, pigs' feet, and silicone suturing pads

Central venous catheter insertion

    Didactic overview via locally developed online module

    Barrier precautions review

    Central venous catheter (CVC) kit setup review

    Task training practice on central-line trainers

    Introduction to ultrasonography guidance

    Formal assessment (multiple choice questions and checklist observation)

Energy sources

    Hands-on practice with bovine electrocautery and ultrasonic coagulator

    Use of device on chicken breasts to simulate OR experience

Surgical biopsy

    Hands-on practice of fine-needle aspiration, core needle biopsy, and incisional/excisional biopsy

    Use of olives imbedded in chicken breasts as simulation

Basics of laparoscopy

    Didactic overview/demonstration of components of laparoscopic equipment

    Pelvic trainer practice in basic drills (rope pass, bean drop, and camera navigation)

Chest-tube insertion

    Didactic overview of closed system one-way valve drainage system

    Hands-on practice in chest-tube insertion in low-tech model (beef ribs overlying IV bag) or cadaver/live porcine model (combined with other procedures)

Surgical airway

    Didactic overview and video demonstration using locally developed content

    Hands-on practice in cricothyroidotomy using cadaver/live porcine model (combined with other procedures)

Airway management

    Hands-on practice in bag-mask ventilation, insertion of oral and nasal airways, placement of laryngeal mask airway, and endotracheal intubation

    Done on full-scale manikin simulators

Stapling techniques

Didactic overview of principles of good anastomoses

Hands-on practice using surgical staplers and foam (gastrointestinal anastomosis staplers, TA staplers, and end-to-end anastomosis staplers)

Splinting

Didactic overview of principles of upper extremity and hand splinting

Hands-on practice on peers

Small group discussions

Common management problems (common calls from floor nurses, common patient questions)

Operative case logging (effective use of ACGME case log system)

Effective documentation

Effective medical-student teaching

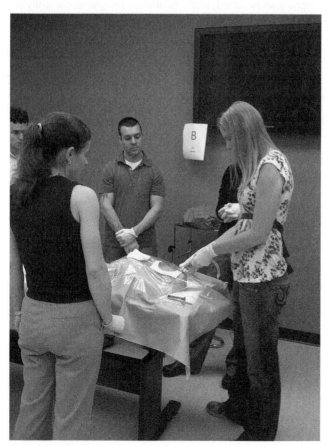

Fig. 1. Learners in the task training room of the Howard and Joyce Wood Clinical Simulation Center at Washington University, Saint Louis.

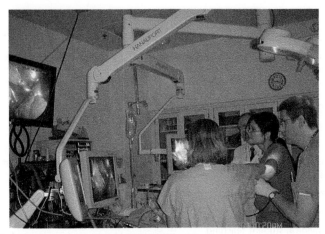

Fig. 2. Resident trainees practicing laparoscopic skills.

including supply lists; recommended reading and learning objectives are among the excellent resources also included. Many residency programs currently use the curriculum in whole or in part. Those programs, such as the one at Washington University, which developed curricula prior to this national resource development, tend to use

---

Box 3
Modules included in phase I of the ACS/APDS National Skills Curriculum

Asepsis and instrument handling

Knot tying

Suturing

Tissue handling, dissection, and wound closure

Advanced tissue handling, flaps, and skin grafts

Urethral and suprapubic catheterization

Airway management

Chest-tube insertion and thoracentesis

Central venous access, arterial lines

Surgical biopsy

Arterial anastomosis

Laparotomy: opening and closure

Principles of bone fixation and casting

Inguinal anatomy

Lower and upper endoscopy

Basic laparoscopic skills

Advanced laparoscopic skills

Handsewn anastomosis

Stapled anastomosis

a combination of the National Curriculum and homegrown modules. Nevertheless, this National Curriculum represents a significant resource, and should aid in the standardization of skills instruction and potential assessment across residency programs.

SIU Model

Many current skills laboratories, including that at Washington University, have borrowed heavily from the forward-thinking curriculum established many years ago at SIU under the leadership of Dr Gary Dunnington. Many of the modules in the curriculum detailed in **Box 2**, as well as in phase I of the ACS/APDS National Curriculum, are modified from the SIU program. An important current component of the program at SIU is the formal verification of proficiency (VOP) that is required of trainees before they are allowed to serve as operating surgeons in the OR.[10] A series of skills-laboratory tasks and virtual procedures are practiced until a level of internally determined proficiency is met. Once this is achieved in practice, trainees are required to submit to formal evaluation of performance in the skills-laboratory setting. Only after a level of proficiency is achieved is the trainee permitted to assume the role of surgeon in the OR. This time- and resource-intensive model surely represents the future of assessment in skills laboratories.

COGNITIVE TASK ANALYSIS/JUDGMENT TRAINING

An important component of skills training that is not specifically addressed in most skills curricula is intraoperative decision making and judgment. In our focused skills training for interns at Washington University, we spend most of our effort ensuring that our learners are adept at basic tasks and skills. However, it has long been recognized that decision making is a critical component in ensuring the successful outcome of an operation.[13] There is an important and growing line of investigation into the question of whether judgment and operative decision making can be taught in skills laboratories. Several studies have shown that, indeed, these skills can be taught and learned in a simulated environment.[14–17] Using cognitive task analysis, the components of an operation that an expert has automated can be broken down and dissected into discrete and teachable components.[14–17] This has been done for several procedures, including laparoscopic Nissen fundoplication, colonoscopy, flexor tendon repair, and percutaneous tracheostomy placement. This strength of skills laboratories needs to be fully realized in the near future; indeed, a recent article has charged the surgical education community with capitalizing on this and incorporating it into surgical training.[18]

LIMITATIONS TO INTENSIVE INTERN SKILLS CURRICULA
Logistics

The limitations to instituting and implementing a full curriculum in simulation for interns and senior students are many and can be daunting. Logistics of scheduling learners to come to the skills laboratory sessions can be difficult because of the patient care responsibilities of interns, their call schedules, and the potential for many trainees to rotate at sites remote from the skills center. With regard to students, coordinating elective schedules during the spring of senior year can be difficult.

Personnel needed to staff skills laboratories can prove costly, but are essential. Given the periodic nature of skills sessions, a full-time individual may not make the most sense; yet, having an individual dedicated to collecting the necessary supplies and orchestrating the session itself is imperative. Space is often a luxury at hospitals and medical schools; thus, having a dedicated space in which to hold these sessions can be difficult to obtain. Ideally, the space would be shared among many user groups, ranging from medical students (undergraduate medical education) to residents/fellows (GME), and even physicians in practice seeking continuing medical education (CME). Many medical schools and hospitals are fortunate to have space that is custom designed and outfitted solely for such sessions, but this is not a necessity. Traditional classrooms can easily be transformed into skills laboratories with minimal effort.

Timing of Training

With regard to scheduling the training sessions, in addition to the aforementioned logistical issues, the optimal timing for skills instruction proximate to operative experience is unknown. It makes intuitive sense that these skills should be taught and practiced when trainees are experiencing a clinical application of the specific skills. That is, residents on a vascular surgery rotation should optimally be learning and practicing their handsewn vascular anastomosis techniques in skills laboratories during the weeks spent on that rotation. The problem for these intensive preparation sessions for interns is twofold: (1) they are typically done with large groups of learners who will be on a variety of clinical rotations; and (2) the actual operative or clinical experience of interns varies widely, and there may not be a clinical opportunity to put the learned skills into actual practice to a significant degree during the sometimes nonoperative or little-operative intern year.

One creative approach to incorporating skills training into residency was recently described by investigators at the University of Washington, Seattle (WA), USA.[19] The residents there spend a dedicated block of time on a rotation specifically designed to protect time for learning and practice in the skills laboratory. Although this solves some problems regarding finding trainee time for learning and practice, the concerns of logistics (teaching few learners frequently vs many at once) and lack of relevance to current clinical rotation persist in this model.

Assessment

As mentioned previously, the intensive intern skills curriculum at Washington University has been in place for 8 years, but assessment is a minor feature. Anecdotal evidence confirms that our experience mirrors that of most skills training programs across the country. The reasons for this are many but there are 3 main barriers, namely, time, lack of standardized instruments, and remediation strategies.

With regard to time, often in short supply is the time required to perform assessments: both individual assessor time (often a surgeon faculty member) and individual trainee time. Getting assessor and trainee together is often logistically difficult because of clinical demands. However, it has been shown that using videotapes of actual operative cases performed by residents is a valid, reliable, and feasible means for assessment in a residency program.[20] In addition, there is a lack of validated and widely available assessment instruments, including agreed-on standardized proficiency standards. Although we work to develop such instruments and standards, it is important to remember that the number of items on the assessment instrument itself is less important than the number of observations.[21] A shorter checklist but more observations of the behavior are important. We also lack a clear course of action for those requiring remediation. Specifically, there is no current standard across residency programs as to when a trainee needs to be proficient in a given procedure (other than on graduation from the program). Further, the current time-based structure of GME (5 clinical years to board eligibility in general surgery) does not lend itself to remediation specifically based on proficiency or competency.

To many of us in GME, these assessment hurdles can be daunting, especially in the face of trying to merely provide a well-organized and efficient skills curriculum. Ideally, some method of VOP similar to the model at SIU should be widely implemented as a first step toward implementation of a full assessment program. Nevertheless, assessment is clearly needed, because it will give our trainees critical information on their performance and areas needing improvement to provide optimal patient care. It is predicted that in the future, formal assessment of technical abilities will be part of the ongoing Maintenance of Certification effort by the American Board of Medical Specialties.[18]

SUMMARY

Skills development during surgical residency would best be served by the acquisition of a solid baseline skills set as early in internship as possible. If this goal is to be accomplished, we believe it is essential that this process be started in the fourth year of medical school, and it should be strengthened and reinforced during the intern year. Indeed, Folse[22] stated more than 10 years ago that "we have failed to use efficiently the fourth year of medical school to prepare our students for entering their residency education", and the Blue Ribbon Committee on Surgical Education from the American Surgical Association has advocated core skills training for medical students preparing for internship as well.[23] Such a process might lessen the demands for intensive "boot camp" type programs during internship and would hopefully enable surgical interns to focus more on patient care and learning operative procedures, and would go a step further toward reducing basic skills development in the OR setting. Students in the fourth year have the time, energy, and motivation to participate in intern preparation courses, which have been shown to enhance skill performance and confidence levels to a significant degree. Furthermore, we would suggest that extending key components of surgical intern skills training to fourth year students should not be overly burdensome, given the mandate for surgical skills programs for all surgical training programs. At a bare minimum, incoming surgical interns should be able to carry out the full range of basic suturing and knot-tying skills at predefined proficiency levels. The time has come for Departments of Surgery including the various surgical specialties to collaborate with Schools of Medicine to provide the necessary personnel, equipment, and other resources that are needed to enhance the critical transition from student/intern to surgical resident.

REFERENCES

1. Tavakol M, Mohaghedgi MA, Dennick R. Assessing the skills of surgical residents using simulation. J Surg Educ 2008;65:77–83.
2. Boehler ML, Rogers DA, Schwind CJ, et al. A senior elective designed to prepare medical students for surgical residency. Am J Surg 2004;187:695–7.
3. Brunt LM, Halpin VJ, Klingensmith MA, et al. Accelerated skills preparation and assessment for senior medical students entering surgical internship. J Am Coll Surg 2008;206:897–907.
4. Hauge LS, Brunsvold ME, Arble EP, et al. M4 Bootcamp: preparing senior students for surgical internship. Oral presentation at the Central Group on Educational Affairs (CGEA) Spring Meeting. Rochester (MN), March 28, 2009.
5. Pierce RA, Tiemann D, Matthews BED, et al. Outcomes of fundamentals of laparoscopic surgery (FLS) skills training for senior medical students entering surgical residency. Surg Endosc 2009;23(S):S332.

6. Peyre SE, Peyre CG, Sullivan ME, et al. A surgical skills elective can improve student confidence prior to internship. J Surg Res 2006;133:11–5.

7. Esterl RM, Henzi DL, Cohn SM. Senior medical student "boot camp" can result in increased self-confidence before starting surgery internships. Curr Surg 2006;63: 264–8.

8. Meier AH, Henry J, Marine R, et al. Implementation of a Web-and simulation-based curriculum to ease the transition from medical school to surgical internship. Am J Surg 2005;190:137–40.

9. Robertson TE, Winslow EJ, Berger L, et al. Specialty specific skills acquisition of incoming post-graduate year one residents. FOCUS on Surgical Education 2006; 23:16–9.

10. Scott DJ, Dunnington GL. The new ACS/APDS skills curriculum: moving the learning curve out of the operating room. J Gastrointest Surg 2008;12:213–21.

11. Williams RG, Dunnington GL, Folse JR. The impact of a program for systematically recognizing and rewarding academic performance. Acad Med 2003;78: 156–66.

12. Duncan JR, Henderson K, Street M, et al. Central venous access: creating and evaluating a simulation-based curriculum. J Grad Med Educ 2010. [Epub ahead of print].

13. DaRosa D, Rogers DA, Williams RG, et al. Impact of a structured skills laboratory curriculum on surgery residents' intraoperative decision-making and technical skills. Acad Med 2008;83:568–71.

14. Peyre SE, Peyre CG, Hagen JA, et al. Laparoscopic Nissen fundoplication assessment: task analysis as a model for the development of a procedural checklist. Surg Endosc 2009;23:1227–32.

15. Sullivan ME, Ortega A, Wasserberg N, et al. Assessing the teaching of procedural skills: can cognitive task analysis add to our traditional teaching methods? Am J Surg 2008;195:20–3.

16. Luker KR, Sullivan ME, Peyre SE, et al. The use of a cognitive task analysis-based multimedia program to teach surgical decision making in flexor tendon repair. Am J Surg 2008;195:11–5.

17. Sullivan MEK, Brown CV, Peyre SE, et al. The use of cognitive task analysis to improve the learning of percutaneous tracheostomy placement. Am J Surg 2007;193:96–9.

18. Bell RH. Why Johnny cannot operate. Surgery 2009;146:533–42.

19. Horvath KD, Mann GN, Pellegrini C. EVATS: a proactive solution to improve surgical education and maintain flexibility in the new training era. Curr Surg 2006;63:151–4.

20. Larson JL, Williams RG, Ketchum J, et al. Feasibility, reliability and validity of an operative performance rating system for evaluating surgery residents. Surgery 2005;138:640–7.

21. Williams RG, Verhulst S, Colliver JA, et al. Assuring the reliability of resident performance appraisals: more items or more observations? Surgery 2005;137: 141–7.

22. Folse JR. Presidential address: surgical education—addressing the challenges of change. Surgery 1996;120:575–9.

23. Debas HT, Bass BL, Brennan MF, et al. American Surgical Association Blue Ribbon Committee report on surgical education: 2004. Ann Surg 2004;241:1–8.

Assessment and Feedback in the Skills Laboratory and Operating Room

Colin Sugden, MRCS*, Rajesh Aggarwal, PhD, MA, MRCS

KEYWORDS

• Assessment • Feedback • Skills laboratory • Operating room

WHY IS ASSESSMENT IMPORTANT?

The term "assessment" describes the final appraisal of an individual or organization's worth and the information gathering process that precedes it. Assessments may establish cutoff points for entry into a period of training, track progress, or ensure standards are adhered to. Historically, our profession has relied on a combination of the subjective opinion of trainers[1] and surrogate markers of performance to determine the competency level of individual surgeons. However, time served and experience, although important, are now known to be weak indicators of skill at best and confounding factors at a team[2] and an institutional level[3] complicate the interpretation of patient outcomes data.

The urgent need for the incorporation of accurate performance assessments into medical training and certification was most noticeably highlighted by the landmark publication of *To Err is Human* in 1998 by the Institute of Medicine in which it was revealed that between 43,000 and 98,000 preventable deaths occur each year in American hospitals. Surgery contributes significantly to this statistic. In the Utah Colorado Medical Practice Study, half of all adverse events experienced by patients who received an operation were believed to be preventable.[4] Accurate and reliable methods with which to accurately determine the competency level of surgical practitioners have now been vigorously pursued and if carefully implemented may make a significant contribution to the quality of patient care in several important ways:

- Selection. The availability of valuable training opportunities in the clinical domain has been reduced in recent years. Candidates in possession of key attributes,

Division of Surgery, Department of Surgery and Cancer, Imperial College London, 10th Floor, QEQM Building, St Mary's Hospital, Praed Street, London, W12 1NY, UK
* Corresponding author.
E-mail address: c.sugden@imperial.ac.uk

Surg Clin N Am 90 (2010) 519–533
doi:10.1016/j.suc.2010.02.009
0039-6109/10/$ – see front matter © 2010 Elsevier Inc. All rights reserved.

surgical.theclinics.com

such as efficient motor learning, are likely to glean the most benefit from exposure to these increasingly limited training opportunities.

- Training. Providing candidates with feedback on their own performance will enable them to strive toward expert benchmarks, moving on to the next stage of training only once proficiency has been reached. Such proficiency-based training enhances the efficiency and quality of training by tailoring the program to the needs of the individual. Underperforming candidates may be identified early in this process and appropriate remedial measures prescribed.
- Certification. Surgery is a rapidly evolving specialty. It is important that new procedures are introduced safely and with minimal risk to patients. Certification will be a crucial step toward fostering public confidence in trainees who are achieving competencies for the first time and experienced practitioners seeking to expand their practice.
- Revalidation. Regular mandatory appraisals of skill are required to identify poor performers early, before patient care is compromised.
- Innovation and research. The ability to standardize operative performance before the commencement of randomized controlled trials of surgical therapy addresses 1 of the most important limitations of previous surgical research. Potential confounding individual and team influences may also be identified and accounted for by the judicious application of repeated performance assessments of each treatment arm.

WHAT NEEDS TO BE ASSESSED?

In the lexicon of surgical educators, performance is said to depend on the successful integration of so-called technical and nontechnical skills. A surgeon's technical skill is deemed to be primarily a function of his or her manual dexterity, and nontechnical skill a function of their decision-making, communication, teamwork, and leadership abilities. Technical proficiency is fundamental to the safe and effective delivery of surgical care. However, many experienced surgeons believe that possession of highly developed nontechnical skill is the true hallmark of a successful surgeon.[5]

TYPES OF ASSESSMENT: SUMMATIVE AND FORMATIVE

This semantic device enables a distinction to be made between assessments on which important decisions are likely to be based and those simply intended to provide supportive feedback to trainees. Summative assessments might determine a candidate's eligibility for entry into a program of training or suitability for progression and as such are typically performed in examination conditions. Formative assessments provide the candidate or their tutor with information about his or her progression, thus promoting efficient learning. Individual weaknesses may be highlighted and addressed, and training may be directed toward achieving predetermined benchmarks.[6]

The terms "summative" and "formative" do not apply to the assessment tool, but rather the way the resulting information is used. This division may not always be a useful one and it is inevitable that occasionally formative and summative assessments will be performed based on data derived from the same assessment procedure. In addition, we believe that formative assessments should be subjected to the same rigorous scientific evaluation as summative assessments to maximize the quality and training efficiency of educational programs.

ASSESSMENT QUALITY
Validity

Performance assessments that have validity in a particular domain can be assumed to provide meaningful and valuable information. Validity can be divided into several categories:

- Face validity is defined as the extent to which the assessment tool resembles the real-life situation. Surgical assessment models with strong face validity include live animal models and high-fidelity virtual reality (VR) simulators. Face validity is typically based on expert opinion gathered using a structured questionnaire.
- Content validity is defined as the extent to which the content of the assessment is appropriate to the situation. Again, this is confirmed by formally canvassing expert opinion.
- Construct validity is the extent to which an assessment tool measures the domain it purports to measure. Construct validity may be assessed in several ways. The most common is to determine its ability to discriminate between novices and experienced candidates.
- Concurrent validity is the level of agreement between the assessment tool in question and another established form of assessment. This is typically assessed by determining the correlation of results obtained by both assessments performed on the same population without any intervening training.
- Predictive validity is the extent to which an assessment tool is able to predict the performance of an individual or group at a future time point or on a different model (sometimes referred to as transfer validity). This is determined by assessing the relationship between either 2 temporally independent assessments or 2 assessments on different models.

Reliability

Reliability refers to the precision of the test, that is, its consistency between assessments and between raters. The reliability of an assessment tool may be assessed in the following ways:

- Retest reliability. Refers to the stability of the test results between multiple assessments. An assessment performed twice on the same subject or group without any intervening training should generate identical results. However, tests are rarely this precise. When an accurate assessment of an individual's performance is required the reliability coefficient between the 2 sets of data should be greater than 0.9. In general, 0.8 is considered to be useful test, 0.5 to 0.8 less so, and less than 0.5 of little use.
- Inter-rater reliability. Applies to observational rating scales. Similar to retest reliability but instead this term refers to the same assessment performed twice by 2 independent assessors. This term may also refer to the level of inter-rater agreement assessed by reliability analysis. 0.8 is considered to be a useful test, 0.5 to 0.8 less so, and less than 0.5 of little use.
- Internal consistency. The correlation between scores in the individual categories of a rating scale or individual simulator-derived parameters is termed the internal consistency of the test. Internal consistency determines whether the individual scores are related and therefore likely to be measuring the same construct.

Feasibility

In order for a valid and reliable assessment regime to be successfully adopted by researchers or program directors it must also be feasible to implement. Despite the description of many reliable and valid measures of surgical performance in recent years, few centers possess comprehensive assessment facilities. Although the reasons for this are complex, it is likely that feasibility issues such as cost and practicality account for much of this discordance. The ideal assessment tool in this regard would be cost-effective, simple to perform, ergonomically attractive, low maintenance, offer flexibility, and not require complex costly installation or experienced members of staff.

Rating scales, an apparently simple method of assessing performance in the skills laboratory and operating room (OR), are only truly valid and reliable if completed post hoc by 2 independent assessors. Multiple assessments of each candidate are also usually desirable, either to chart progression, or to account for the characteristic variation in case mix encountered in an OR environment. The demand this places on the valuable time of experienced faculty members is too great for many institutions, thereby rendering their use unfeasible.

The training of junior surgeons is a considerably burdensome undertaking from a financial perspective. A recalcitrant approach to the adoption of potentially expensive new technologies until their cost-effectiveness has been clearly demonstrated is, therefore, understandable. The case for more frequent and more innovative assessments must be made, in cost terms, on the potential for a well-implemented assessment regime to enhance training efficiency and improve patient safety.[7,8] Much work is needed before clear evidence of this kind will be available; large studies designed to track multiple effects from training efficiency to patient outcome measures will need to be performed.

BUILDING AN ASSESSMENT PROCEDURE

The components of a surgical performance assessment are largely dependent on the environment or context in which the assessment occurs. In turn, assessment tools are dependent on the surgical model with which they are aligned (**Box 1**).

ASSESSMENT ENVIRONMENT
Operating Room

Advantages
In many ways the most desirable context for an assessment of surgical performance to take place is the OR. As previously discussed, the effective delivery of surgical

---

Box 1
Components of a surgical assessment

Context (A): operating room
  1. Model: real patients
  2. Assessment tools: dexterity parameters, rating scales

Context (B): laboratory
  1. Model: human/animal cadaveric, live animal, synthetic, basic tasks, virtual reality, augmented reality
  2. Assessment tools: number of procedures, final product analysis, dexterity parameters, rating scales

treatments is dependent on individual technical performance, decision-making skills, and the ability to function well as a member of the OR team.[9] This complex challenge faced by practicing surgeons differs dramatically from the artificial, nonthreatening setting of the skills laboratory. Assessments performed in the skills laboratory are now capable of reaching a high standard of validity and reliability. However, patient care is delivered exclusively in the OR environment. Therefore, assessment programs designed to enhance care delivery and improve patent safety may be rooted in the skills laboratory environment but cannot exist without effective measures of OR performance.

Anatomic variation, difficult pathology, equipment problems, and physiologic disturbance are all common in the OR but difficult to simulate elsewhere. Face and content validity issues common to laboratory-based simulation assessments may limit the degree of engagement with the tasks experienced by assessment candidates. Lack of immersion in the simulation may alter behavior and affect performance.[10] The OR environment maximizes engagement, motivation, and focus, thereby enhancing the scientific value of the assessment regime.

Disadvantages

Although the model and context provided by the OR are in many ways ideal, assessment in this environment is a challenging undertaking. The scientific value of assessments may be restricted by variations in case mix and the influence of OR staff or assistants.[11] Furthermore, options for objective assessment of performance in the OR are comparatively limited and suffer from feasibility issues, such as poor ergonomics in the case of motion analysis and, in the case of video-based rating, the considerable time investment required. Live rating of performance, although more feasible, is weakened by the potential for rater bias and therefore cannot be considered reliable. Subjects may also alter their performance in response to being visibly assessed, an observation known as the Hawthorne effect.

It is never acceptable to compromise patient safety in the course of performance assessments. To this end, training and assessment outside the OR must occur for candidates to demonstrate proficiency in a controlled environment.[12] Therefore, OR assessment is likely to be used either to assess senior practitioners or to assess trainees who have successfully completed a regime of laboratory assessments.

Skills Laboratory

Advantages

The laboratory environment, although artificial, is nonthreatening and controllable. Novice or junior surgeons will inevitably make mistakes as they progress through the various stages of skill acquisition. In the laboratory setting such mistakes may be identified and learned from without any threat to patient safety; errors here harm the trainee's assessment alone.

It is important that, as far as possible, the assessment tool measures only the desired construct: the individual surgeon's performance.[6] The absence of OR staff or assistants helps to isolate the performance of an individual surgeon in a way not possible in the context of the OR. Simulation models are also, by their very nature, standardized and repeatable. Administered to large populations, this form of assessment allows for peer group comparisons to be made and benchmarks to be set. Data obtained in this way may be used formatively by individual candidates engaged in training and by faculty to identify poor candidates for remedial action and strong candidates for fast-track programs. Such data are also likely to be used as a means to conduct internal audits at an institutional level.

A wide range of assessment tools are available in the skills laboratory. The feasibility of assessment using dexterity analysis devices and audiovisual recording equipment is enhanced in the absence of ergonomic restraints inherent to the OR. VR simulation, a model now gaining popularity in simulation laboratories, brings with it the potential for enhanced realism, flexibility, and many unique assessment advantages.[13] VR-derived metrics go beyond simple dexterity analysis and can therefore provide candidates with more detailed instantaneous feedback on dexterity and procedure quality.

Disadvantages
The laboratory setting lacks the contextual cues, immediacy, and interaction of a real OR. Candidates are likely to feel less immersed in the assessment task and may lack motivation or alter their behavior.[10] Laboratory assessments also generally focus on specific techniques and narrow sets of skills. Although there are undoubtedly advantages to this approach, proficiency in this setting cannot be accepted as a surrogate for effective real-world performance. Simulation of whole complex procedures is possible using animal models and VR simulators, but these facilities are currently limited to specialist centers and therefore not available to most trainees.

SIMULATION MODELS

Effective laboratory assessment depends on the availability of suitable simulation models. Many are available, each with their own benefits and limitations. Fidelity and feasibility are the main factors that determine the suitability of a simulation model for use in a particular assessment.

Physical

Live animal
Live animal models offer a level of fidelity unmatched by any other form of simulation model. Techniques such as the ligature of major vessels, tissue hemostasis, and dissection in natural planes may all be assessed with a greater degree of accuracy in the presence of live perfused organs than on any other model. Despite this, animal models cannot claim to accurately represent human anatomy. Some come close, but even the commonly used porcine model lacks important anatomic features such as a sigmoid mesocolon.

There has been a trend in recent years toward the use of image-based endoscopic and percutaneous techniques that lend themselves well to all forms of simulation from live animal to VR. However, open surgery is much more challenging to simulate and as a result relies much more heavily on human, animal, and synthetic models.

Live animal laboratories are generally expensive to run because of the cost of anesthetic equipment, experienced staff, and the requirement to purchase, house, care for, and dispose of the animals used. Many important ethical issues must be considered (a discussion of which is beyond the scope of this review) when contemplating the use of live animal simulation models, particularly as more sophisticated VR devices become available, and for this reason the practice is proscribed in the United Kingdom.

Cadaveric Models

Human
Human cadaveric models are used infrequently because of cost and lack of availability. They have the advantage of being anatomically correct, although tissues do not bleed and there is no respiration. As previously mentioned, although VR will almost certainly be the dominant simulation model adopted by endoscopic surgery, open surgery is likely to rely on physical models for some time to come.

Animal

Used frequently by technical skills courses, animal cadaveric tissue models such as the porcine gallbladder are generally considered to display a high degree of anatomic accuracy. In common with other cadaveric tissues, however, manipulation and dissection can lack realism as the handling properties differ from those of live tissue and, crucially, no bleeding occurs when tissues are cut. In addition, cadaveric models placed inside a laparoscopic box are artificially separated from the important anatomic structures with which they are usually in close proximity. Disengagement and unsafe instrument use are potential consequences of this situation.

Synthetic Models

Procedural

High-quality models are available. These are relatively cheap and avoid the ethical issues that live or cadaveric tissue models present. However, the dissection planes are generally unrealistic and the tissues do not bleed when cut.

Basic tasks

Basic tasks such as stacking sugar cubes and peeling grapes in a laparoscopic box trainer allow novices to become accustomed to the fulcrum effect and acquire a degree of laparoscopic dexterity.

Virtual Reality

Currently available VR devices range from low-fidelity abstract models such as the MIST-VR[14] to complex high-fidelity simulators incorporating techniques from laparoscopic,[15] endovascular,[16] and sinus surgery[17] to gastrointestinal endoscopy[18] and arthroscopy.[19] The most important advantage that VR simulation has over other less costly models is the ability to provide immediate detailed feedback to the candidate. This includes measures of dexterity such as path length and number of movements as well as task-specific parameters such as torque, insertion force, and mucosal visualization in the case of endoscopy and volume of contrast and fluoroscopy time in the case of endovascular simulation (**Fig. 1**). In addition, error rates measured by the simulator provide a form of immediate objective data regarding the quality of the procedure.

Patient File	15/15 09-22-09 13:52:25
Total procedure time	00:24:55
Total fluoroscopy time	00:07:32
Interventional procedure(s)	3
Number of guide wires used	3
Number of Dx catheters used	2
Time to obtain Dx images of arch	00:01:17
Time to position guide/sheath proximal to bifurcation	00:02:20
The duration of time the postdilation balloon was opened	00:00:10

Fig. 1. Endovascular metrics.

VR simulators allow the user to predetermine the difficulty of the assessment exercise enabling the same simulator to fulfill several different assessment roles. In addition, although VR simulators are costly to purchase, their maintenance costs are significantly lower than comparable forms of physical simulation. Simulation laboratories using live or cadaveric animal models must be staffed by skilled faculty members and must continually replenish their specimen stocks. VR models on the other hand may be used on multiple occasions without any additional maintenance cost and provide immediate objective feedback to the candidate, reducing the requirement for staffing during formative assessments.

ASSESSMENT TOOLS

Regardless of what environment the assessment is performed in or what surgical model is used, a range of assessment tools are available. These range from imprecise surrogate measures such as the number of procedures performed to more reliable and objective measures such as dexterity parameters and observational rating scales (**Table 1**).

Observational Rating Scales

Informal human assessment of performance is the oldest and probably the most common form of surgical assessment. However, it is also one of the most unreliable. It is natural for surgeons to critique their own performance and for tutors to provide informal feedback to their trainees; this is a fundamental component of the traditional Halstedian apprenticeship model. Unfortunately the scientific reliability and therefore the ultimate value of this type of assessment is low, leaving significant room for improvement.[1] Observational rating scales endeavor to objectify this process by providing specific guidance on what areas of the procedure to assess and a structured scoring system with which to do so. The simple addition of rating scales to human assessments significantly enhances their reliability and validity.

Global Rating Scales

Global rating scales aim to measure components of effective surgical performance common to many procedures such as respect for tissues and instrument handling.

Table 1
Comparison of assessment tools

Assessment Method	Technical Skill		Nontechnical Skill		Feasibility	
	Validity	Reliability	Validity	Reliability	OR	Laboratory
Surrogate markers						
Patient outcomes	Low	Low	Low	Low	High	N/A
No. of procedures performed	Low	Low	Low	Low	High	High
Human assessment						
Self-assessment	Low	Low	Low	Low	High	High
Unstructured opinion	Low	Low	Low	Low	High	High
In training assessments	Low	Low	Low	Low	High	High
Rating scales (live)	High	Moderate	High	Moderate	Low	Moderate
Rating scales (video)	High	High	High	High	Low	Moderate
Objective parameters						
Dexterity metrics	High	High	N/A	N/A	Low	High

The scale used to score the Objective Structured Assessment of Technical Skill (OSATS) devised by Martin and colleagues[20] includes 7 performance items, each of which is allocated a mark from 1 to 5. Marking is further standardized by the anchoring of specific descriptors to marks 1, 3, and 5. This scale was validated on live animal and benchtop models for inclusion in the OSATS examination and has subsequently been successfully validated for the assessment of a wide range of technical procedures by other research groups.[21–24] Inter-test and inter-rater coefficients are consistently found to be around 0.7 or more suggesting that they are a reliable objective measure of generic technical performance.[25]

Procedure-specific Scales

Global rating scales are successful measures of the overall quality of surgical procedures however, by their very nature, they are unable to identify at which specific part of the operation a deficiency was present. Procedure-specific scales address this problem. Scales that enable raters to highlight steps that are performed incorrectly have a clear application as formative assessment tools.[26] A trainee in possession of this information may enhance the efficiency of their training by concentrating on a subset of relevant laboratory-based tasks rather than practicing the whole procedure.

The scale devised and validated by Eubanks and colleagues[27] for laparoscopic cholecystectomy breaks the procedure down into its component parts, each of which is assigned a numeric value to be awarded on successful completion. A set of errors are also defined and are assigned a score in a similar fashion. The raw score and error score are combined resulting in a final procedural score. This scale demonstrated good validity and reliability (r = 0.74–0.96). However, unfortunately many such scales have failed to match the scientific value of their generic counterparts.[25,27]

Rating Scales of Nontechnical Performance

A revised version of the NOnTECHnical Skills (NOTECHS) scale, developed to assess the nontechnical skills necessary for safe performance in the aviation industry, has been developed for use in the context of surgical performance.[28] The revised scale measures 5 domains including: communication and interaction, situation awareness and vigilance, cooperation and team skills, leadership and managerial skills, and decision-making. Each domain consists of 4 to 5 items allocated a score between 1 and 6.

MOTION TRACKING

Motion-tracking devices allow manual dexterity to be objectively measured during the course of a real procedure or on a physical model in the skills laboratory. The ability to objectify the rating of operative performance and provide immediate feedback to the candidates is otherwise only available in the realm of VR simulation. An example of one such system is the Imperial College Surgical Assessment Device (ICSAD) and ROVIMAS motion-tracking software.[29] The ICSAD uses an Isotrack II electromagnetic device to track the position of sensors on the back of the surgeons hands in the x, y and z axis. ROVIMAS software, running on a laptop computer, enables the recorded data to be quantified and reported instantly. The system also has the capacity to record synchronized video of the procedure to be sent for post hoc observational rating. The construct validity of ICSAD has been demonstrated in the laboratory on benchtop models[30] and in the OR environment on laparoscopic cholecystectomy.[31]

Comparison of Assessment Tools

Research has been performed in our department to determine the relationship between motion analysis, video-based rating and a variety of observational rating scales in the assessment of laparoscopic cholecystectomy.[25,32] Global rating scales have performed consistently well, yielding strong validity and reliability results. Procedural scales and checklists on the other hand performed poorly displaying low precision and failing to differentiate experienced practitioners from novices.[25] Results from the ICSAD motion analysis system correlated well with global rating scales and was a valid assessment of the most challenging part of the operation: Calot triangle dissection.[32] See **Table 1** for a comparison of the reliability, validity, and feasibility of assessment tools.

Evolution of Laboratory Assessment

There is much to recommend the use of a traditional nonthreatening laboratory environment particularly for the assessment of junior trainees or novices. However, as already discussed, assessments performed in this setting measure only a subset of the skills required for successful performance in a real OR. For a truly rigorous in vitro assessment of surgical performance, candidates must be required to perform well technically while at the same time exercising good judgment and communicating well with the theater team.

Simulated Operating Suite

In an attempt to achieve a more rigorous training and assessment environment, our department has invested in a simulated operating suite (SOS) that aims to replicate a real OR with as much realism as possible (**Fig. 2**). The SOS (designed exclusively for research, training, and assessment purposes) is equipped with a fully functional operating table, suction machines, diathermy, laparoscopic stack, and operating room lights. Real surgical instruments and materials such as dressings and sutures are also available. A moderate fidelity anesthetic simulator recreates cardiovascular and respiratory complications and a high-fidelity laparoscopic simulator recreates a wide range of procedures from laparoscopic cholecystectomy to gastric bypass and sigmoid colectomy. The theater team is made up of experienced actors who allow a predetermined sequence of events to play out, thus standardizing the assessment.

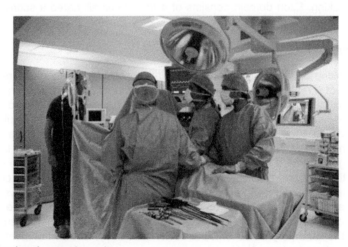

Fig. 2. Simulated operating suite.

Live observational assessments of technical and nontechnical skill may be performed from a control room or performed post hoc using recordings made by discreetly placed video cameras and microphones. Assessments may be augmented by dexterity parameters derived from ICSAD or by parameters generated by the VR simulator.

Challenging pressured conditions are common in the real OR. The use of trained actors and carefully developed scenarios enables candidates skills to be truly stretched in a controlled, standardized, and repeatable fashion, successfully bridging the gap between assessments in the OR and laboratory environment.

In Situ Simulation

An alternative, potentially more cost-effective approach to contextual simulation is the use of empty theater or clinical space to stage simulation-based assessments at weekends and out of hours. In situ simulation requires no initial financial outlay and maximizes the use of currently available resources. It also successfully bridges the gap between laboratory and OR assessment by placing the simulation scenario in an actual clinical environment. Although it may seem to be an ideal solution, the limitations of this approach become apparent when compared with a purpose-built simulated operating suite. These include the lack of sufficient recording facilities in most conventional ORs, the absence of a control room for live observational assessment, and the inherently unpredictable nature of opportunistically commandeering unused clinical space for educational purposes.

NEW TECHNOLOGIES

New technologies currently under investigation with the potential to provide a biomarker of effective skill acquisition or even expertise are near-infrared spectroscopy (NIRS) and eye tracking.

NIRS

NIRS is a noninvasive, functional, neuroimaging technique that works by shining near-infrared light through the scalp into the underlying cortical tissue.[33] Scattered reflections are then detected by a set of low light-sensitive photodiode detectors and tissue perfusion is inferred from the differential absorption spectra of oxygenated and deoxygenated hemoglobin. The use of cerebral perfusion patterns as a surrogate for cortical activation by indirect neuroimaging techniques such as fNIRS and functional magnetic resonance imaging (fMRI) is justified because of the close relationship known to exist between neuronal activation and cerebral blood flow.[34]

The principal advantages of fNIRS over fMRI in the assessment of surgical performance are its portability, tolerance of movement, and lack of intrusive noise. Work is ongoing to identify the neural substrates underlying surgical task performance and the learning process involved. Existing research in this area is promising; prefrontal cortical behavior during a surgical knot-tying task has been shown to vary according to years of surgical experience,[35] and neuroplastic changes in the brain have been seen to occur in response to the practice of a surgical task.[36] Both these findings support the potential future use of this technique as a biomarker of technical proficiency and effective skill acquisition. However, more research is required.

Eye Tracking

Human eyesight lacks a uniform visual response. Outwith the foveal region of the retina, which represents around 1 to 2 degrees of visual angle, acuity drops off sharply. Therefore, our ability to appreciate a scene is heavily dependent on the rapid voluntary eye movements (saccades) that direct our fovea toward areas of interest and on that gaze being maintained for long enough to be consciously appreciated (fixations). Eye tracking is achieved by using distinguishable features of the eyes including the limbus, pupil, and corneal reflection to determine the position of fixations and the order in which they occur. A commonly used method involves shining infrared light onto the eyes and tracking the corneal and lens reflections known as Purkinje reflections.[37]

Eye movements, referred to as a microcosm of the brain,[38] may help elucidate the thought processes of an expert surgeon and the image features they rely on to perform an operation. Identification of optimum search patterns may help identify inefficient or atypical behavior from which judgments about the experience level and decision-making ability of an individual may be derived. For example, differences in use of two-dimensional information during the performance of a laparoscopic task can be used to compare the performance of individual surgeons.

SURGICAL INNOVATION

Surgically delivered care is rarely static and indeed most therapies undergo a continual process of adaptation and evolution in response to the demand for a higher standard of patient care. Unfortunately new surgical procedures, particularly in the early phase of their development, introduce an element of instability or unpredictability to the patient-treatment pathway. For a period of stability to be reached, the new technique must be carefully developed and learned and its efficacy must be fully established. Minimally invasive surgery, now considered a successful innovation, serves as an example of the potential for a promising new technology to lead to unacceptable morbidity and mortality on its introduction.[39]

That attempts to enhance the standard of care we provide in the future may put patients, to whom we owe a duty of care, at risk, is an unwelcome and perhaps unnecessary paradox. Laboratory training and assessment allow techniques to be learned in a controlled environment and performance to be standardized across the treatment arms of a randomized controlled trial thereby addressing an important criticism leveled at prior surgical research.[40] Patient specific VR simulators, a technology already in existence, may be used to generate a model of the patients anatomy, pathology, and physiology enabling the procedure to be rehearsed beforehand.[41] Potential problems may be identified in the safety of the skills laboratory and standardized strategies may be agreed on to help overcome them entirely.

Treatments that are considered efficacious may also now be adopted in a similarly structured manner, consisting of an initial laboratory training and assessment phase followed by a period of OR-based assessment and culminating finally in full certification once competence has been achieved.

SUMMARY

The wide range of possible combinations of context, model, and assessment tools currently available allow assessments to be tailored to meet the needs of selection and certification procedures, training curricula, and surgical research teams. As already discussed, it is important that valid and reliable assessment tools are aligned with a model and context appropriate to the competency of the individual. The application of these principles to the assessment of an advanced laparoscopic procedure **(Fig. 3)** illustrates how this can be achieved. Assessment begins in the safety of the skills laboratory where candidates must demonstrate proficiency, first on a range of basic techniques and finally on the whole procedure, before entering the OR. The use of a wide range of metrics including dexterity parameters and rating scales of performance enhances the scientific and training value of the assessment procedure. Crucially, assessments culminate in the OR where, candidates able to demonstrate proficiency progress to the next phase of their training and those who do not attend for a further assessment in the skills laboratory. This mechanism functions to preserve patient safety and enhance training efficiency by enabling candidates to address specific deficiencies in the controlled environment of the skills laboratory.

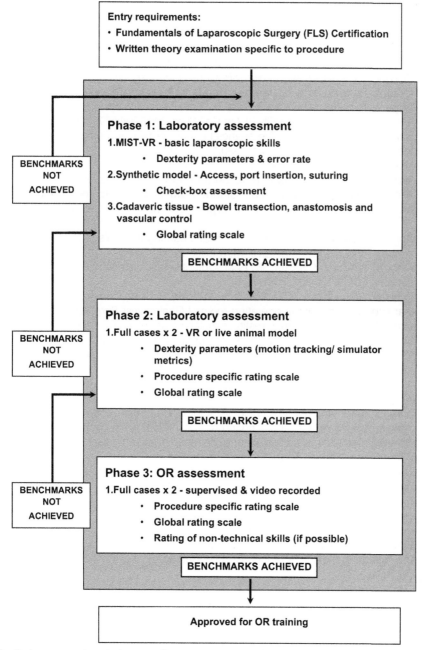

Fig. 3. Laparoscopic anterior resection assessment program.

REFERENCES

1. Reznick RK. Teaching and testing technical skills. Am J Surg 1993;165:358–61.
2. Schaefer HG, Helmreich RL, Scheidegger D. Safety in the operating theatre–part 1: interpersonal relationships and team performance. Curr Anaesth Crit Care 1995;6:48–53.
3. Westrum R. Social factors in safety-critical systems. In: Redmill R, Rajan J, editors. Human factors in safety critical systems. Oxford: Butterworth-Heinemann; 1997. p. 233–56.
4. Studdert DM, Thomas EJ, Burstin HR, et al. Negligent care and malpractice claiming behavior in Utah and Colorado. Med Care 2000;38:250–60.
5. Baldwin PJ, Paisley AM, Brown SP. Consultant surgeons' opinion of the skills required of basic surgical trainees. Br J Surg 1999;86:1078–82.
6. Aggarwal R, Grantcharov TP, Darzi A. Framework for systematic training and assessment of technical skills. J Am Coll Surg 2007;204:697–705.
7. Bridges M, Diamond DL. The financial impact of teaching surgical residents in the operating room. Am J Surg 1999;177:28–32.
8. Haluck RS, Satava RM, Fried G, et al. Establishing a simulation center for surgical skills: what to do and how to do it. Surg Endosc 2007;21:1223–32.
9. Greenberg CC, Regenbogen SE, Studdert DM, et al. Patterns of communication breakdowns resulting in injury to surgical patients. J Am Coll Surg 2007;204:533–40.
10. Kneebone RL, Nestel D, Moorthy K, et al. Learning the skills of flexible sigmoid-oscopy - the wider perspective. Med Educ 2003;37(Suppl 1):50–8.
11. Moorthy K, Munz Y, Sarker SK, et al. Objective assessment of technical skills in surgery. BMJ 2003;327:1032–7.
12. Scott DJ, Dunnington GL. The new ACS/APDS Skills Curriculum: moving the learning curve out of the operating room. J Gastrointest Surg 2008;12:213–21.
13. Grantcharov TP. Is virtual reality simulation an effective training method in surgery? Nat Clin Pract Gastroenterol Hepatol 2008;5:232–3.
14. Wilson MS, Middlebrook A, Sutton C, et al. MIST VR: a virtual reality trainer for laparoscopic surgery assesses performance. Ann R Coll Surg Engl 1997;79:403–4.
15. Aggarwal R, Crochet P, Dias A, et al. Development of a virtual reality training curriculum for laparoscopic cholecystectomy. Br J Surg 2009;96:1086–93.
16. Van Herzeele I, Aggarwal R, Choong A, et al. Virtual reality simulation objectively differentiates level of carotid stent experience in experienced interventionalists. J Vasc Surg 2007;46:855–63.
17. Edmond CV. Impact of the endoscopic sinus surgical simulator on operating room performance. Laryngoscope 2002;112:1148–58.
18. Moorthy K, Munz Y, Jiwanji M, et al. Validity and reliability of a virtual reality upper gastrointestinal simulator and cross validation using structured assessment of individual performance with video playback. Surg Endosc 2004;18:328–33.
19. Howells NR, Gill HS, Carr AJ, et al. Transferring simulated arthroscopic skills to the operating theatre: a randomised blinded study. J Bone Joint Surg Br 2008;90:494–9.
20. Martin JA, Regehr G, Reznick R, et al. Objective Structured Assessment of Technical Skill (OSATS) for surgical residents. Br J Surg 1997;84:273–8.
21. Swift SE, Carter JF. Institution and validation of an observed structured assessment of technical skills (OSATS) for obstetrics and gynecology residents and faculty. Am J Obstet Gynecol 2006;195:617–21 [discussion: 621–3].

22. Friedman Z, Katznelson R, Devito I, et al. Objective assessment of manual skills and proficiency in performing epidural anesthesia – video-assisted validation. Reg Anesth Pain Med 2006;31:304–10.
23. van der Heide PA, van Toledo-Eppinga L, van der Heide M, et al. Assessment of neonatal resuscitation skills: a reliable and valid scoring system. Resuscitation 2006;71:212–21.
24. Moorthy K, Munz Y, Dosis A, et al. Bimodal assessment of laparoscopic suturing skills: construct and concurrent validity. Surg Endosc 2004;18:1608–12.
25. Aggarwal R, Grantcharov T, Moorthy K, et al. Toward feasible, valid, and reliable video-based assessments of technical surgical skills in the operating room. Ann Surg 2008;247:372–9.
26. Beard JD, Choksy S, Khan S, et al. Assessment of operative competence during carotid endarterectomy. Br J Surg 2007;94:726–30.
27. Eubanks TR, Clements RH, Pohl D, et al. An objective scoring system for laparoscopic cholecystectomy. J Am Coll Surg 1999;189:566–74.
28. Sevdalis N, Davis R, Koutantji M, et al. Reliability of a revised NOTECHS scale for use in surgical teams. Am J Surg 2008;196:184–90.
29. Datta V, Mackay S, Mandalia M, et al. The use of electromagnetic motion tracking analysis to objectively measure open surgical skill in the laboratory-based model. J Am Coll Surg 2001;193:479–85.
30. Torkington J, Smith SG, Rees BI, et al. Skill transfer from virtual reality to a real laparoscopic task. Surg Endosc 2001;15:1076–9.
31. Smith SG, Torkington J, Brown TJ, et al. Motion analysis. Surg Endosc 2002;16:640–5.
32. Aggarwal R, Grantcharov T, Moorthy K, et al. An evaluation of the feasibility, validity, and reliability of laparoscopic skills assessment in the operating room. Ann Surg 2007;245:992–9.
33. Strangman G, Boas DA, Sutton JP. Non-invasive neuroimaging using near-infrared light. Biol Psychiatry 2002;52:679–93.
34. Roy CS, Sherrington CS. On the regulation of the blood-supply of the brain. J Physiol 1890;11:85–158. 17.
35. Leff DR, Orihuela-Espina F, Atallah L, et al. Functional near infrared spectroscopy in novice and expert surgeons–a manifold embedding approach. Med Image Comput Comput Assist Interv 2007;10(Pt 2):270–7.
36. Leff DR, Orihuela-Espina F, Atallah L, et al. Functional prefrontal reorganization accompanies learning-associated refinements in surgery: a manifold embedding approach. Comput Aided Surg 2008;13:325–39.
37. Yang GZ, Dempere-Marco L, Hu XP, et al. Visual search: psychophysical models and practical applications. Image Vis Comput 2002;20:291–305.
38. Carpenter RH. Frontal cortex. Choosing where to look. Curr Biol 1994;4:341–3.
39. Cuschieri A. Whither minimal access surgery: tribulations and expectations. Am J Surg 1995;169:9–19.
40. Ergina PL, Cook JA, Blazeby JM, et al. Challenges in evaluating surgical innovation. Lancet 2009;374:1097–104.
41. Cates CU, Patel AD, Nicholson WJ. Use of virtual reality simulation for mission rehearsal for carotid stenting. JAMA 2007;297:265–6.

FLS and FES: Comprehensive Models of Training and Assessment

Melina C. Vassiliou, MD, MEd[a],*, Brian J. Dunkin, MD[b],
Jeffrey M. Marks, MD[c], Gerald M. Fried, MD[d]

KEYWORDS

- Fundamentals of Laparoscopic Surgery
- Fundamentals of Endoscopic Surgery • GOALS • GAGES
- Simulation • Technical skills • Assessment • Competence

FLS

The Fundamentals of Laparoscopic Surgery (FLS) program was developed by surgeons, educators, and administrators, under the leadership of the Society of American Gastrointestinal and Endoscopic Surgeons (SAGES). The impetus to create this curriculum came from the need to safely introduce laparoscopic techniques into clinical practice and from the demand to demonstrate basic competence in the application of this new technology.[1] In the early years of laparoscopy, some surgeons integrated this technique into their practices after cursory weekend courses or animal laboratories. However, an increase in bile duct injuries and other complications occurred with the first laparoscopic cholecystectomies.[2] This critical issue of patient safety was the initial driver for the FLS effort. Around the same time, the concept of simulation in medicine was also gaining popularity, especially in light of restricted resident work hours and limited operating-room resources. It was entirely logical to take the learning process for new procedures and technologies out of the operating room and into a safe, controlled environment.

[a] Department of Surgery, McGill University Health Centre, McGill University, 1650 Cedar Avenue, #L9.518, Montreal, Quebec H3G 1A4, Canada
[b] Department of Surgery, The Methodist Hospital, Weill Cornell Medical College, 6550 Fannin Street, Suite 1661A, Houston, TX 77030, USA
[c] Department of Surgery, University Hospitals, Case Medical Center, 11100 Euclid Avenue, Mail Stop 5047, Cleveland, OH 44106, USA
[d] Department of Surgery, McGill University Health Centre, McGill University, 1650 Cedar Avenue, #L9.309, Montreal, Quebec H3G 1A4, Canada
* Corresponding author.
E-mail address: melina.vassiliou@mcgill.ca

Surg Clin N Am 90 (2010) 535–558
doi:10.1016/j.suc.2010.02.012   surgical.theclinics.com

The vision for the FLS program was created in the late 1990s among some of the leaders in the SAGES organization. They recognized the need for the program to meet the highest educational standards, especially if the intent was to demonstrate a basic level of competence. The program was designed as a tool to teach the fundamental knowledge and technical skills considered by experts to be necessary for safe and effective laparoscopic surgery. The unique feature of FLS is the associated metrics that measure the outcome of the educational intervention and that can verify learning and establish a level of basic competency. This article describes the components of FLS and the rigorous validation process that helped it to become an important certification program for surgeons and one of the requirements to be eligible for the American Board of Surgery (ABS) examination. Because of this solid foundation, FLS has been used as the basis for educational research to improve our understanding of how best to learn and teach these essential skills. The second part of this article describes the Fundamentals of Endoscopic Surgery (FES) program, which is currently in the final stages of development, and which SAGES has modeled after FLS.

THE FLS PROGRAM

The mission of the program is stated on the FLS Web site (http://www.flsprogram.org/):

To provide surgical residents, fellows and practicing surgeons an opportunity to learn the fundamentals of laparoscopic surgery in a consistent, scientifically accepted format; and to test cognitive, surgical decision-making, and technical skills, all with the goal of improving the quality of patient care.

The curriculum is not procedure or discipline specific. It includes general concepts and elements of decision making that are related to the equipment, technology, and physiology of laparoscopic surgery and can be used to teach and assess gynecologists, urologists, general surgeons, and other surgical subspecialists.[3–5] The objectives of the program can also be found on the FLS homepage and are shown in **Table 1**. The program is offered to practicing surgeons who use laparoscopy and to trainees in accredited surgical training programs.

Since 2005, FLS has been a joint program of SAGES and the American College of Surgeons (ACS) and it is managed by a committee of members from both

Table 1 Objectives of the FLS program
To improve the quality of care received by patients undergoing laparoscopic surgery
To set minimum standards for basic cognitive and technical skills used in performing laparoscopic procedures
To provide surgeons practicing laparoscopy with standardized didactic information on the fundamentals of laparoscopic surgery and a tool to assist in development of judgment and manual skills
To create an objective quantifiable measure to assess knowledge, judgment, and manual skills in basic laparoscopic surgery
To make available to hospitals and institutions a validated tool to measure the knowledge and skills fundamental to the performance of laparoscopic surgery
To improve the quality of care received by patients undergoing laparoscopic surgery

organizations. In addition, FLS is one of the modules included in the ACS-APDS (Association of Program Directors in Surgery) technical skills curriculum that has been recently introduced.[6] As mentioned, the ABS has included FLS certification as a requirement to be eligible to write the qualifying examination (http://home. absurgery.org/default.jsp?certgsqe; accessed on November 13, 2009). Although not yet required by the Royal Australasian College of Surgeons, FLS certification is strongly endorsed by the association.

PROGRAM DESCRIPTION AND COMPONENTS

The FLS program includes teaching and assessment components. The Web-based study guides consist of didactic modules, patient scenarios, and technical skills explanations organized into content areas. Multiple educational modalities, including video and high-quality photographs, are used to illustrate important concepts. The modules include Preoperative Considerations, Intraoperative Considerations, Basic Laparoscopic Procedures, Postoperative Care and Complications, and Manual Skills Practice (**Table 2**). Each module ends with practice questions and the text and the questions can be printed for review. In the past, this material was available in CD format, but it is now all Web-based. The online program is practical and also offers the possibility to track how learners use the program, how much time they spend on each module, and how they perform on the practice questions. This program can be linked with a learning management system and may be useful for program directors and course supervisors. The assessment of this didactic material is done in the form of a 90-minute multiple-choice examination of 75 questions. The computer-based test must be taken in a proctored setting at designated testing centers. It includes standard multiple-choice questions as well as case-based scenarios, and sometimes asks the examinee to interpret digital images.

Table 2 Web-based FLS modules	
Preoperative considerations	1. Laparoscopic equipment 2. Energy sources 3. Room setup 4. Patient selection and preoperative assessment
Intraoperative considerations	1. Anesthesia and patient positioning 2. Pneumoperitoneum establishment and trocar placement 3. Physiology of pneumoperitoneum 4. Exiting the abdomen
Basic laparoscopic procedures	1. Diagnostic laparoscopy 2. Biopsy 3. Laparoscopic suturing 4. Hemorrhage and hemostasis
Postoperative care and complications	1. Postoperative care 2. Access injuries 3. Pneumoperitoneum 4. Surgical injury 5. Procedural complications
Manual skills instruction and practice	1. Training exercises 2. Data analysis

The second part of the teaching component focuses on manual skills and consists of a detailed description with videos of 5 tasks performed in a box trainer. A curriculum for practice is recommended, based on proficiency goals derived by expert laparoscopists, and is described in detail later in this article.[7,8] These performance goals differ slightly from the passing scores required in the test situation, but are practical and, if achieved consistently, almost guarantee a passing score on the examination. Trainees are encouraged to practice in a distributed fashion and to review the videos frequently to see how they are progressing. Intermittent proctoring and focused feedback by an expert surgeon or trained laboratory technician can also be helpful to learners and should be available on request or according to a schedule.[9] Trainees are free to practice the skills as frequently as they like, and they can arrange to take the examination when they think they are ready. FLS is also a valuable tool for junior residents to practice their skills before going to the operating room, and can be used as a way to maintain the skills of surgeons or residents who have already been certified.

The FLS technical skills curriculum is performed in a standard box trainer with a built-in camera that is connected to a monitor (not included, **Fig. 1**). The kit also contains a set of instruments and disposable supplies (**Fig. 2**). The entire box, except for the monitor, can be collapsed into a practical carrying case for easy transport. The manual skills component includes 5 tasks modeled after the original program developed by Derossis and colleagues,[10] and previously referred to as the McGill Inanimate System for the Training and Evaluation of Laparoscopic Skills (MISTELS; **Table 3**, **Figs. 3–7**). The 5 tasks include peg transfer, precision cutting, placement of a ligating loop, and suturing using extracorporeal and intracorporeal knot tying. The tasks are scored for efficiency and precision, and each task has a predetermined cutoff time. The scores are normalized and are equally weighted. A higher score indicates superior performance. The tasks described are the same for the practice curriculum and the supervised certification examination, which must be taken in designated test centers and scored by trained proctors. More detailed information about each of the tasks can be found on the FLS Web site (http://www.flsprogram.org/).

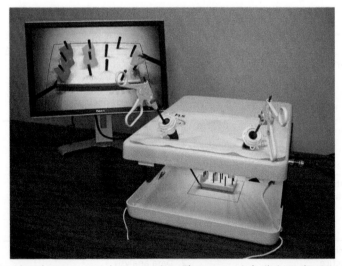

Fig. 1. FLS trainer box connected to a monitor. The camera is built into the top of the box. (*Reprinted from* the Society of American Gastrointestinal and Endoscopic Surgeons; with permission.)

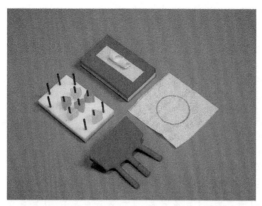

Fig. 2. Disposables and props used in the FLS trainer box. (*Clockwise from the pegboard*) Penrose drain and block, circle pattern on gauze for pattern cutting, and foam appendages for ligating loop. (*Reprinted from* the Society of American Gastrointestinal and Endoscopic Surgeons; with permission.)

FLS VALIDATION PROCESS
Manual Skills Component

The first step in the creation of the manual skills program involved expert review of videotaped procedures with the intent to identify key components that are unique to laparoscopy, and that differentiate it from open surgery. A list of items was generated, which then served as a foundation for the development of the box-trainer tasks (**Table 4**). The FLS trainer box is simple, inexpensive, and standardized. As described later, the metrics have been extensively validated and meet the necessary standards for high-stakes evaluations.

Reliability of the Metrics

Reliability is concerned with the consistency of the test results and can be measured in different ways. However, a reliable test is not necessarily a valid test. Validity implies the extent to which the test approximates or measures reality. Reliability standards must be met to proceed with validation testing, but a reliable test is not itself a valid test.

The FLS metrics were examined for inter-rater and test-retest reliability. The internal consistency of the 5 tasks was also evaluated. High inter-rater reliability suggests that different evaluators will rate the same performance in a similar manner, and that the variability in scores between individuals is related to variability in skills and not between evaluators. Inter-rater reliability for the FLS metrics was 0.998, which is considerably more than the required 0.8 for high-stakes assessments.[11] Test-retest reliability implies that outcomes are consistent when the same trainee is evaluated on different occasions without a change in skill level. The test-retest reliability for total FLS score was 0.89.[11] An adequate test should also show internal consistency between test items, suggesting that they are all measuring some aspect of a general construct, such as laparoscopic skills. This criterion is estimated using the Cronbach α, which was 0.86 for the FLS tasks. The internal consistency could not be improved with the elimination of any of the tasks, indicating that they are not redundant. Scores on each individual task correlated highly with total scores.[11]

Table 3
Tasks and descriptions for the FLS, manual skills

Task	Equipment/Cutoff (s)	Description
Peg transfer (**Fig. 3**)	Maryland dissectors, pegboard, 6 objects 300	Lift the 6 objects with a grasper first in the nondominant hand and transfer the object to the dominant hand. Then, place each object on a peg on the opposite side of the board. Once all 6 pegs have been transferred, the process is reversed. This exercise tests eye-hand coordination, ambidexterity, and depth perception
Precision cutting (**Fig. 4**)	Maryland dissector, endoscopic scissors, 4×4 gauze, alligator clips 300	One hand should be used to provide traction on the gauze. Start cutting from an edge of the gauze. A penalty is assessed for deviation from the line demarcating the circle. This exercise requires the use of both hands in a complimentary manner
Placement and securing of ligating loop (**Fig. 5**)	Grasper, endoscopic scissors, large clip, 1 pretied ligating loop or endoloop, 1 foam organ with appendages 180	Place a pretied ligating loop or endoloop around a tubular foam appendage on the provided mark. A penalty will be assessed if the knot is not secure and for any distance that the tie misses the mark. This skill can be used, for example, in the operating room for ligation of the appendix at its base or for securing a dilated cystic duct
Simple suture with extracorporeal knot (**Fig. 6**)	Needle drivers (or choice of 1 needle driver and 1 grasper), knot pusher, suture of 90–120 cm, endoscopic scissors, Penrose drain with marked targets, suture block 420	Place a simple stitch through 2 marks in a longitudinally slit Penrose drain. Tie the suture extracorporeally, using a knot-pushing device. Tie the knot tightly enough to close the slit in the drain. At least 3 square throws are required to ensure that the knot will not slip under tension. A penalty is applied for any deviation of the needle from the marks, any gap in the longitudinal slit in the drain, and a knot that slips when tension is applied to it. If the drain is avulsed from the block, a score of zero will be applied
Simple suture with extracorporeal knot (**Fig. 7**)	Two needle drivers, suture of 15-cm length, endoscopic scissors, suture block, Penrose drain with marked targets 600	Place a suture precisely through 2 marks on a Penrose drain, then tie using an intracorporeal knot. Place at least 3 throws that must include 1 double throw and 2 single throws on the suture. Ensure that the knots are square and will not slip. Between each throw, the needle must be transferred to the other hand. Skills required include proper placement of the needle in the needle holder, needle transferring, suturing skills, and knot tying. This is a more complex task, incorporating several skills including depth perception, eye-hand coordination, ambidexterity, and transferring skills

Reprinted from the Society of American Gastrointestinal and Endoscopic Surgeons; with permission.

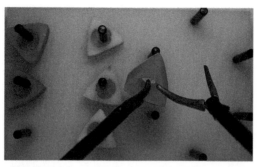

Fig. 3. Peg transfer. (*Reprinted from* the Society of American Gastrointestinal and Endoscopic Surgeons; with permission.)

VALIDITY OF FLS MANUAL SKILLS METRICS AND SIMULATOR
Face and Content Validity

Face validity is derived from expert opinion. Face validity should not be confused with resemblance to real life, which is referred to as fidelity. Some simulators use gamelike environments, which do not look like the real task, but experts consider them to represent many of the important skills that are required for the actual skill. A test has good face validity if a group of experts agree that, at face value, it seems to measure what it intends to measure. Content validity is also acquired from the opinions of content experts. It is slightly different in that it is concerned with whether or not the test includes all of the important aspects of a given skill; the comprehensiveness of the test items. It is also established by consulting a group of experts.

The manual skills component of FLS has face and content validity according to a global rating scale given to experts about the credibility of the metrics and the content of the tasks. In addition, the process by which it was developed confers an inherent validity because it was developed by content experts with the goal of simulating important laparoscopic skills. Laparoscopic surgeons assembled a list of 14 skills required to safely perform surgery using this technology. Participants of the manual skills tasks were asked how many of the skills were represented in the 5 tasks, and most considered 11 to be incorporated in the FLS program.[12] The skills not included were safe use of the electrosurgical unit, cannulation, and initial trocar placement. This knowledge is part of the Web-based didactic program, and the FLS committee is currently considering the addition of cannulation and camera navigation tasks to the simulator.

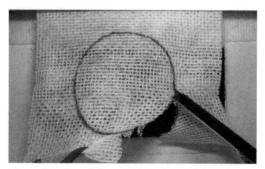

Fig. 4. Precision cutting. (*Reprinted from* the Society of American Gastrointestinal and Endoscopic Surgeons; with permission.)

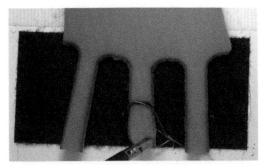

Fig. 5. Placement and securing of ligating loop. (*Reprinted from* the Society of American Gastrointestinal and Endoscopic Surgeons; with permission.)

Construct and External Validity

Construct validity needs to be evaluated when an objective assessment of the concept to be measured does not exist, and a known surrogate must be used. In this case, the surrogate would be level of training. Expert laparoscopic surgeons would be expected to outperform novices if the simulator and metrics were truly measuring laparoscopic skills. The FLS manual skills metrics were able to show significant differences in performance between novice, intermediate, and expert surgeons when they were examined according to training, experience (self-reported), or self-assessment of competence.[13,14] A subset of the larger cohort was assessed over time, and scores in the simulator increased as the participants garnered additional clinical expertise.[10] Fraser and colleagues[15] created receiver operator curves using level of experience (a known variable) to define novice (first- and second-year surgical residents) and experienced (chiefs, fellows, and attending laparoscopic surgeons) groups. The FLS scores for these groups were used to create receiver operator curves that would indicate a cutoff score to help differentiate surgeons that were competent or incompetent in the basic skill set required for laparoscopy. The passing total score was selected to provide optimal sensitivity, specificity, and positive and negative predictive values (all were >0.80),[15] and was set at a normalized score of 270.

External validity assesses the generalizability of the test results and its applicability to different situations or individuals. The greater the diversity of the study population, the more generalizable the results tend to be. The FLS manual skills program was tested by a group of 215 surgeons from 5 countries around the world.[13]

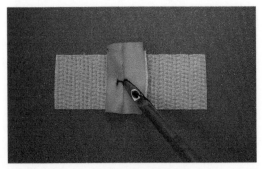

Fig. 6. Simple suture with extracorporeal knot. (*Reprinted from* the Society of American Gastrointestinal and Endoscopic Surgeons; with permission.)

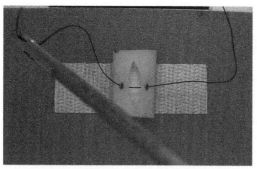

Fig. 7. Simple suture with intracorporeal knot. (*Reprinted from* the Society of American Gastrointestinal and Endoscopic Surgeons; with permission.)

Criterion Validity

Criterion validity is divided into 2 areas: concurrent and predictive. Concurrent validity asks whether simulator performance correlates with performance on other related measures of the skill set. MISTELS scores were shown to correlate with the technical skills assessment from in-training evaluations [16] and performance of laparoscopic procedures in an animal laboratory.[17]

Predictive validity asks whether performance on the simulator will predict future performance in the clinical environment. Predictive validity is the most powerful type of validation for simulation, and shows the value of the simulator as a predictor of technical competence. To show predictive validity, an objective, reliable, and valid measure of operative performance is needed. In 2005, the Global Operative Assessment of Laparoscopic Skills (GOALS) was developed and validated during dissection of the gallbladder from the liver bed.[18] GOALS is a 5-item scale with anchors at 1, 3, and 5 that was developed specifically to measure basic laparoscopic skills in the clinical environment (**Fig. 8**). The items include depth perception, bimanual dexterity, efficiency, tissue handling, and autonomy, and the maximum total score is 25. The correlation between MISTELS scores and GOALS scores within 2 weeks of each other was 0.81.[13] McCluney and colleagues[19] subsequently evaluated a larger group of surgeons in the FLS simulator and in the operating room using GOALS. Multivariate analysis found FLS score to be an independent predictor of operative performance. An FLS score of 70 (corresponding to a total score of 350) predicted a GOALS score of 20 or greater (range of experienced surgeons).[19]

Table 4
Fundamental differences between open and laparoscopic surgery
Monocular vision/limited depth perception
Magnification
Fixed access through a trocar/decreased degrees of freedom
Fulcrum effect
Long instruments that amplify tremor and provide decreased tactile feedback

Reprinted from the Society of American Gastrointestinal and Endoscopic Surgeons; with permission.

Date: _____   Operator: _____
Attending: _____   Level of Training: _____

Global Operative Assessment of Laparoscopic Skills – GOALS

GLOBAL RATING SCALE - GRS

1. Depth Perception
Score:

1. Constantly overshoots target, wide swings, slow to correct.
2.
3. Some overshooting or missing of target, but quick to correct
4.
5. Accurately directs instruments in the correct plane to target

2. Bimanual Dexterity
Score:

1. Uses only one hand, ignores non-dominant hand, poor coordination between hands
2.
3. Uses both hands, but does not optimize interaction between hands
4.
5. Expertly utilizes both hands in a complimentary manner to provide optimal exposure

3. Efficiency
Score:

1. Uncertain, inefficient efforts, many tentative movements, constantly changing focus or persisting without progress
2.
3. Slow, but planned movements that are reasonably organized
4.
5. Confident, efficient and safe conduct, maintains focus on task until it is better performed via an alternative approach

4. Tissue Handling
Score:

1. Rough movements, tears tissue, injures adjacent structures, poor grasper control, grasper frequently slips
2.
3. Handles tissues reasonably well, minor trauma to adjacent tissue (i.e. occasional unnecessary bleeding or slipping of the grasper)
4.
5. Handles tissues well, applies appropriate traction, negligible injury to adjacent structures

5. Autonomy
Score:

1. Unable to complete entire task, even with verbal guidance
2.
3. Able to complete task safely with moderate guidance
4.
5. Able to complete task independently without prompting

Total   /25

Fig. 8. GOALS, used for intraoperative assessment.

RELIABILITY AND VALIDITY OF THE COGNITIVE ASSESSMENT

The creation of the knowledge-based assessment was an iterative process that was guided by expert surgeons on the SAGES FLS committee, in consultation with educational psychologists and statisticians. The questions were vetted for relevance and importance by surgeons from a variety of backgrounds and then reviewed by the committee (face and content validity). Poorly performing questions were revised or eliminated, and ultimately 2 examinations were prepared for field testing.[14] Eight centers in North America participated in the process. Demographic information about level of training, laparoscopic experience, and self-ratings of competence in laparoscopic surgery was gathered. The validity of the cognitive examination was established by finding significant differences in scores based on laparoscopic experience, while controlling for level of training. The test was shown to measure differences in laparoscopy-specific knowledge as opposed to overall general surgery knowledge (level of training). Self-ratings of competence in laparoscopy correlated positively with cognitive test scores.[12] Internal consistency between the multiple-choice and scenario-based questions was 0.60, indicating that they measure a related concept, but that they are not measuring exactly the same aspects. The internal consistency of merged cognitive test items was 0.81.[14]

FLS AS A TRAINING PROGRAM

As described earlier, the validated metrics for the manual skills component of FLS make it an outstanding summative measure of technical competence. However, to be an effective formative tool, a simulator must have an associated curriculum to help trainees efficiently acquire the necessary skills. Work in this area is still ongoing. Ritter and Scott[7] used the FLS tasks to establish proficiency benchmarks for trainees to use during practice. They defined target performances, allowable errors, and reproducibility criteria for each of the tasks (**Table 5**). The metrics are simplified so that trainees can assess their own performance without the need for a trained proctor.[7] This curriculum was then applied to true novices (medical students) who were also asked to record the number of repetitions needed to achieve the established proficiency goals. The students had access to a proctor and to the manuals skills video. They were able to achieve the proficiency levels for 96% of the 5 tasks, and all of them achieved a passing score on the post-test FLS manual skills examination. The mean time required was 9.7 hours, and a mean of 119 repetitions (total of all tasks) were needed to complete the curriculum. The average cost per student of consumable materials for this training was $143.10.[8] There are many ongoing projects using 1 or more of the FLS skills to characterize learning curves,[20,21] determine skill degradation and maintainenance,[22–24] and better understand the ideal interval for distributed simulator practice.[25] The FLS tasks have also been used to understand the attentional demands of learning a new skill, and the concept of automaticity as it applies to technical skills.[26,27]

FLS SIMULATOR PRACTICE IMPROVES OPERATING-ROOM PERFORMANCE

The true test of the effectiveness of the FLS manual skills program as a training program is whether the skills acquired and measured in the simulator transfer to the operating room. Sroka and colleagues[28] recently conducted a randomized controlled trial examining the effects of training using the FLS proficiency-based curriculum described by Ritter and Scott[7] on operating-room performance as measured by GOALS. The FLS-trained group achieved the proficiency goals and improved

Table 5
Proficiency-based curriculum for FLS manuals skills

Task	Allowable Errors	Proficiency Time (s)	No. of Repetitions Required
Peg transfer	No dropped pegs outside the field of view	48	2 consecutive + 10 nonconsecutive
Pattern cut	All cuts within 2 mm of the line	98	2 consecutive
Ligating loop	Up to 1 mm accuracy area, no knot insecurity	53	2 consecutive
Extracorporeal suture	Up to 1 mm accuracy area, no knot insecurity	136	2 consecutive
Intracorporeal suture	No model avulsion	112	2 consecutive + 10 nonconsecutive

Data from Ritter EM, Scott DJ. Design of a proficiency-based skills training curriculum for the Fundamentals of Laparoscopic Surgery. Surg Innov 2007;14:107; Scott DJ, Ritter EM, Tesfay ST, et al. Certification pass rate of 100% for fundamentals of laparoscopic surgery skills after proficiency-based training. Surg Endosc 2008;22:1887.

significantly (increased by 6.1 ± 1.3, $P<.01$) in the operating room compared with the control group whose GOALS scores remained unchanged (increased by 1.8 ± 2.1, $P = .47$).[28] After 2.5 hours of supervised practice, and 5 hours of individual, deliberate practice, the simulator group, composed of first- and second-year residents, performed at the level of third- and fourth-year residents in a previous study.[19] They acquired skills in the simulator in 7.5 hours that they may otherwise have acquired during 1 or 2 years of residency training. These results provide powerful support for the value of the FLS manual skills program in improving operating-room performance.

FLS IN THE DEVELOPING WORLD

A group from Toronto recently conducted a 3-day FLS course in an underserved area in Botswana. Only 2 surgeons among the 20 trainees passed the cognitive and manual skills assessments to obtain certification.[29] After their visit, the group left the FLS equipment behind and conducted a study in which surgeons from Botswana were proctored weekly from Toronto via telesimulation and compared with a control group of surgeons who had access to the equipment and videos without proctoring. The telesimulation group outperformed the control group by achieving FLS scores almost twice as high.[30] In addition, all of the surgeons achieved the FLS certification passing rate for the manual skills compared with 38% in the control group. This finding represents an exciting and cost-effective way to teach surgeons in remote areas using the FLS platform.

FLS CONCLUSION

The FLS program has gained momentum in the past several years. As mentioned earlier, it is now a joint SAGES-ACS program and included in the ACS-APDS curriculum. In addition, Covidien, through a large educational grant, is supporting the FLS program to allow all programs in North America to purchase an FLS trainer box. This program also provides vouchers for all graduating residents and laparoscopic surgery fellows to become FLS certified.[31] To date, more than 3000 vouchers have been provided throughout North America. There are 39 FLS test centers in the United States, 3 in Canada, and several in the Australian continent.

Surgeons in the Harvard system were the first to participate in a malpractice carrier–sponsored FLS course. The 37 participants were motivated to take the course for several different reasons, including directive from chief/chairman, to improve didactic knowledge, to improve manual skills, the $500 incentive offered by the carrier, the belief that FLS would become a standard (like Advanced Trauma Life Support [ATLS] or Advanced Cardiac Life Support [ACLS]), because it was free, or for reasons of Continuing Medical Education (CME) credits.[32] This is the first record of financial incentives being offered by a malpractice carrier for FLS certification.

FES

Many of the same issues that prompted the development of FLS are apparent in the training of competent flexible endoscopists in the fields of gastroenterology and gastrointestinal (GI) surgery. The importance of these skills for surgeons is rapidly increasing as less-invasive methods to treat GI disease are developed. In parallel with this, the Residency Review Committee (RRC) for surgery recently increased the number of flexible endoscopic procedures required of surgical trainees.[33] Case numbers have long been used as a surrogate for procedural competency, and flexible endoscopy is no exception. Other surrogate measures such as polyp detection rates, procedural time, and cecal or pyloric intubation rates have also been used. However, none have been shown to be reliable or valid measures of competence.[34–36] This problem is similar in many ways to the challenges that were raised when laparoscopic surgery was first introduced in the 1980s. In response to the need for an objective way to teach and assess the knowledge and skills required to perform basic flexible endoscopy, members of SAGES began to discuss the possibility of developing a flexible GI endoscopy program, similar to FLS, that could serve as a benchmark for physicians of all specialties.[13] Through this discussion, FES was born. This article describes the development and validation of the didactic and manual skills components of the FES program to date, which has been influenced heavily by the lessons learned during the development of FLS. At the time of preparation of this article, the program is still being developed and validated, with the intention to launch the program by April 2010.

THE VISION

FES was envisioned as a curriculum to teach and evaluate the fundamental knowledge and skills required to perform basic upper endoscopy and colonoscopy. It will include didactic material in Web-based format, an online written examination, and a hands-on skills test on a simulator. The entire examination will be less than 2 hours, and will, through a rigorous validation process, aim to provide objective evidence that the examinee who attains a passing score possesses the knowledge and skills required to perform basic flexible endoscopy.

To be eligible to participate in the FES program, individuals will be required to meet minimum training criteria. For surgeons, the trainee will have to have completed a flexible endoscopy rotation and be in at least the second year of training, and GI fellows will be eligible after the first year of their fellowship. FES is being designed by surgical endoscopists, colorectal surgeons, gastroenterologists, and individuals with expertise in educational psychology.

THE DEVELOPMENT PROCESS

The first discussions about FES occurred in 2005. Subsequent to that meeting, the leadership of SAGES formally endorsed the program, established an FES Task Force, and arranged for start-up funding and administrative support. During the next 6 months, FES Task Force members were selected, an outline for the didactic material was created, and investigators were assigned to content chapters. In January 2006, an FES retreat was conducted during which a comprehensive literature review of all computer-generated and non–computer-generated flexible endoscopy simulators was performed. At that time, the FES didactic chapters were also vetted, and a deconstructed task list of the manual skills required to perform flexible endoscopy was formulated as the basis for the manual skills evaluation. Two subcommittees were then created: one focused on editing the didactic material and developing a written examination, and the other on creating a hands-on skills testing platform for flexible GI endoscopy.

The FES Written Examination

SAGES collaborated with an online secure testing consultant with expertise in creating validated high-stakes examinations to design the didactic component of FES. With the guidance of this consultant, a test definition document was developed that defined the scope of the examination, and a survey was drafted to assess the test document content and to weight each content area, similar to the FLS process. The survey was distributed to general surgeons, colorectal surgeons, and gastroenterologists.

Based on the definition document and the survey, a comprehensive test objectives outline was formulated to specify the exact content of the written FES examination and reflecting the weighted importance of each area by indicating the number of questions assigned to each topic.

This outline was then used as a guide for designing the questions. Multiple question-writing sessions were conducted to ensure the accuracy and congruency of each question. Based on the goal of a 90-minute examination containing 75 questions, it was determined that at least 225 questions (3 times the desired 75) were needed to have a sufficient bank to randomize to each examination after the validation process. Surgeons and gastroenterologists at all levels of training, at multiple β-test sites, and during scientific meetings are evaluating the written examination. Once sufficient numbers are obtained, the data will be analyzed to detect and exclude poor-performing questions and then to establish acceptable pass and fail rates, similar to the way FLS was designed.

Didactic Material

The FES didactic program includes Web-based content similar to a flexible endoscopy textbook to help learners acquire the knowledge that is important for the performance of safe and effective upper endoscopy and colonoscopy. An outline of the content chapters is shown in **Table 6**. Each chapter was reviewed by expert endoscopists for accuracy of content and appropriate breadth and depth, and then edited by 1 of 2 editors assigned to the FES project. SAGES then hired a Web-based learning content and proficiency expert to transform the didactic material into an online format with high-quality illustrations and pictures.

Hands-on Skills Test

In July 2006 another retreat was held to focus on the development of the hands-on skills component of FES. During this meeting, expert surgical endoscopists defined the skills required to perform basic and safe flexible endoscopy (**Table 7**). This list of skills was then used as the basis for designing and evaluating potential testing and learning platforms. Regarding the platform, it was hoped that an inexpensive, off-the-shelf simulator could be modified to meet the needs of the program. However, after a thorough review of existing technology, it became clear that no such platform existed. A request for proposals was submitted, and, after a lengthy process including a simulation fair, it was determined that a computer-generated platform would best

Table 6
List of technical skills required for flexible GI endoscopy

1. Scope navigation
   Tip deflection
   Scope traversal
   Torque
   Use of 2-handed technique
2. Loop reduction
3. Retroflexion
4. Traversing a sphincter
5. Management of insufflation
6. Mucosal evaluation
7. Targeting

Reprinted from the Society of American Gastrointestinal and Endoscopic Surgeons; with permission.

Table 7 Fundamentals of Endoscopic Surgery (FES) didactic content (abbreviated)	
Technology and equipment	Characteristics of endoscopes Equipment setup Trouble shooting Equipment care
Patient preparation	Informed consent Anesthesia risk assessment Prophylactic antibiotic therapy Management of anticoagulation
Anesthesia/conscious Sedation/monitoring/ recovery	Monitoring Conscious sedation Recovery Alternative anesthesia Unsedated endoscopy
Upper endoscopy	Indications/contraindications and surveillance/ screening Patient positioning/room setup Performance of diagnostic esophagogastroduodenoscopy Complications prevention/recognition/correction Normal anatomy Pathology recognition
Lower GI endoscopy	Indications/contraindications and surveillance/ screening Patient position/room setup Performance of diagnostic colonoscopy Normal anatomy Pathology recognition
Endoscopic retrograde cholangiopancreatography (ERCP)	Indications/contraindications and surveillance/ screening Patient position/room setup Performance of diagnostic ERCP Complications prevention/recognition/correction Normal anatomy Pathology recognition Interventions: tissue sampling, sphincterotomy, stone removal, relief of obstruction
Endoscopic therapies	Hemostasis-variceal/nonvariceal Polypectomy Dilation/stent Foreign-body removal Enteral access Combined laparoendoscopic procedures

Reprinted from the Society of American Gastrointestinal and Endoscopic Surgeons; with permission.

suit the needs of the FES skill set. Although such a platform is expected to have a higher price point than originally anticipated, it has several distinct advantages. First, flexible endoscopy equipment is not required, because it uses a proprietary endoscope that does not need to be cleaned or reprocessed. Second, the test can be administered with Web support to standardize administration and eventually eliminate the need for an on-site expert proctor. Third, an electronic platform allows for centralized collation of results with secure reporting and easy dissemination of software upgrades. Fourth, the manufacturers of virtual reality (VR) GI endoscopy platforms voiced a commitment to developing a desktop version that would be significantly more affordable than existing VR training platforms. After a careful selection and negotiation process, a partnership was formed between SAGES and Simbionix (Simbionix Ltd, Israel; manufacturers of the GI Mentor II; **Fig. 9**) to create the hands-on skills component of FES.

THE FES PROGRAM

FES will be a validated program to teach and evaluate the knowledge and skills required to perform basic flexible endoscopy, the first of its kind for this skill set. It comprises 3 elements: (1) Web-based didactic material, (2) a 75-question multiple-choice examination to verify understanding of the material, and (3) a hands-on test of basic flexible GI endoscopy skills. The program will be administered as follows:

Learners will be given access to the Web-based FES content and allowed to review the material at their own pace. When learners are ready, they can register to take the FES examination. The written examination will be performed on a secure Web connection, but administered in a proctored environment. Ninety minutes will be allotted to complete 75 questions, and the results will be electronically reported to SAGES. The final step is the hands-on test. It consists of 5 separate modules administered on the Simbionix GI Mentor II platform. Because of the cost of this platform, it is envisioned that the test will initially be given at regional testing centers around the world. Eventually, the goal is to develop a desktop testing platform, which could be more easily distributed to individual training programs. The 5 testing modules are currently in the final phases of development, and are as follows:

1. Module 1. Navigation (traversal, tip deflection, and torque). The module requires the endoscopist to navigate through a simulated colon by advancing the scope using torque and tip deflection. It is necessary to use 2-handed scope manipulation (1 hand on the deflection wheels; the other on the scope shaft) to successfully complete the task. On screen, the examinee advances through a simulated colon while trying to avoid touching the surrounding walls. There are floating targets

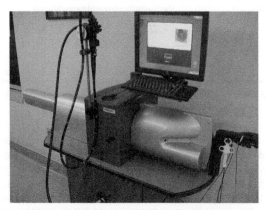

Fig. 9. Simbionix GI Mentor II (Simbionix Ltd, Israel). (*Reprinted from* Simbionix; with permission.)

pointing at different angles, and the operator needs to manipulate the scope within the lumen to line up the viewfinder on the screen with the target (**Fig. 10**).

2. Module 2. Loop reduction. This module requires the trainee to reduce random loops that are created as they advance through the colon. Each loop differs in anatomic configuration and level of difficulty. The testee will see and feel paradoxic movement of the scope in a simulated colon and will not be able to advance without loop reduction (**Fig. 11**).

3. Module 3. Upper GI endoscopy with retroflexion, sphincter traversal, and use of insufflation. The simulated environment consists of the sectional anatomy of the upper GI tract including the esophagus, stomach, pylorus, and first portion of the duodenum. The testee must pass the endoscope into and through the stomach to locate the pylorus. The pylorus is then traversed using a combination of tip control and insufflation, and a target is located in the proximal duodenum. The endoscope is then brought back into the stomach and insufflation and retroflexion are used to identify targets on the incisura and in the cardia. The task is completed by straightening the endoscope, evacuating insufflation, and pulling back into the esophagus (**Fig. 12**).

4. Module 4. Mucosal evaluation. The testee must thoroughly evaluate the colonic mucosa and identify targets using scope control and insufflation. The exercise begins with the endoscope in the cecum, and requires a careful mucosal inspection during scope withdrawal (**Fig. 13**).

5. Module 5. Targeting. The simulation portrays the sectional anatomy of the lower GI tract. While advancing the endoscope, the testee must identify a target and deliver a biopsy forceps to its center without colliding with the visceral wall. Target position is randomized. The biopsy tool must be reintroduced into the working channel for each target (**Fig. 14**).

VALIDATING THE FES EXAMINATION

The implications of such a high-stakes examination, as with the FLS program, are so important that the components must meet the most rigorous standards of reliability

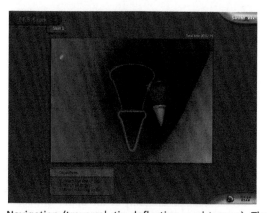

Fig. 10. Module 1. Navigation (traversal, tip deflection, and torque). The module requires the testee to navigate through a simulated colon by advancing the scope and using torque and tip deflection. On screen the testee travels inside a colon trying to avoid touching the surrounding walls. When the trainee reaches a target, the endoscope must be torqued and deflected to line up the viewfinder on the screen with the target. (*Reprinted from* Simbionix; with permission.)

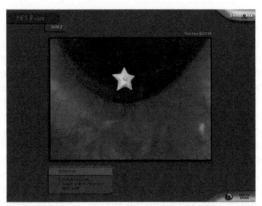

Fig. 11. Module 2. Loop reduction. This module requires the trainee to reduce random loops. The loops differ in anatomic configuration and level of difficulty. On screen, the testee will see paradoxic movement of the scope and will not be able to advance without loop reduction. (*Reprinted from* Simbionix; with permission.)

and validity. The reliability and validity of the FES written examination is being established through the iterative process described earlier. The hands-on skills test is also currently undergoing reliability and validity testing to ensure, as far as possible, that those who pass the examination are, at the least, competent to perform basic flexible endoscopy and to interpret the results of their findings. The manual skills validation process will be briefly described later.

Reliability

Reliability refers to the consistency of the test. It must result in similar outcomes when scored by different evaluators (inter-rater reliability) and must be consistent when the

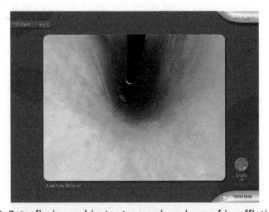

Fig. 12. Module 3. Retroflexion, sphincter traversal, and use of insufflation. The simulated environment consists of the sectional anatomy of the upper GI tract including the esophagus, stomach, pylorus, and first portion of the duodenum. The testee must pass the endoscope into the stomach to locate the pylorus. The pylorus is then traversed using a combination of tip control and insufflation and a target is located in the proximal duodenum. The endoscope is then brought back into the stomach and a combination of insufflation and retroflexion is used to identify targets on the incisura and in the cardia. (*Reprinted from* Simbionix; with permission.)

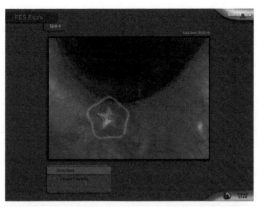

Fig. 13. Module 4. Mucosal evaluation. The testee must thoroughly evaluate the colonic mucosa and identify as many targets as possible using scope control and insufflation. The exercise begins with the endoscope in the cecum and requires a careful mucosal inspection during withdrawal. (*Reprinted from* Simbionix; with permission.)

same trainee is evaluated on different occasions without a change in skill (test-retest reliability). It should also be internally consistent, suggesting that individual items on a test are all measuring some aspect of a general construct, such as flexible endoscopy in this case. Once the reliability of the outcome measure of a simulator is established, validity can be investigated. The reliability testing for FES is currently underway, but will resemble the design used to assess reliability for FLS metrics. The results will be analyzed using intraclass correlation coefficients and the internal consistency of the simulated tasks will be assessed using the Cronbach α.

Validity

Validity can be evaluated in different ways, as was shown with the FLS process. Different types of validity can, together, provide support that the outcome of the

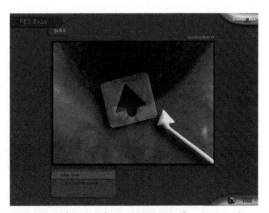

Fig. 14. Module 5. Targeting. The simulation portrays the sectional anatomy of the colon. While advancing the endoscope, the testee must identify a target and deliver a biopsy forceps to its center without colliding into the side walls. The position of targets is randomized. The biopsy tool must be reintroduced into the working channel for each target. (*Reprinted from* Simbionix; with permission.)

test is a true representation of the actual skill or knowledge of the individual. The FES program will be subjected to validity testing similar to FLS and including face, content, construct, external, and criterion validity.

Face and Content Validity

The FES simulator was developed by expert endoscopists who clearly defined the skill set that needed to be respresented in the simulated tasks. They worked closely with Simbionix to create the simulator modules, which went through several iterations before the final version was accepted. The first versions were evaluated at the learning center during SAGES meetings and by selected members of the FES Task Force in their own institutions. This process ensures the face and content validity of the manual skills component of FES.

Construct and External Validity

In this case, because there is no established measure of competence, known groups can be used to establish the truthfulness of the test. For example, expert endoscopists would be expected to outperform novices if the test is truly measuring endoscopic skills. FES is currently undergoing rigorous known groups construct validity testing in a multiinstitutional international trial.

External validity assesses the generalizability of the test results and its applicability or validity to different situations or individuals. The FES program will be validated in different sites around the world, and will include participants from surgical and GI specialties.

Criterion Validity

Criterion validity includes concurrent and predictive validity. Concurrent validity asks whether performance on the simulator mirrors performance in real life. Predictive validity asks whether performance on the simulator predicts future performance. As with the FLS process, predictive validity is the Holy Grail of simulation assessment because it establishes that performance on the simulator correlates with performance in the real clinical environment. Data are still being gathered and analyzed, but the goal is to be able to show that a passing FES score will be a reliable benchmark for competence in flexible endoscopy. FES scores will also help to objectively define a physician's skill set better than current reliance on procedure numbers.

To prove that a simulation platform has predictive validity, there must be a reliable and valid measure of clinical performance. For FLS, the intraoperative tool (GOALS) was developed after the simulator. No such measurement tool was available when the FES project was started so the FES Task Force developed the Global Assessment of Gastrointestinal Endoscopic Skills (GAGES). GAGES is a global assessment tool that can be used to measure technical skills in the real clinical environment (**Figs. 15** and **16**). GAGES-Upper Endoscopy and GAGES-Colonoscopy have been shown in a multicenter trial to be reliable and valid tools to measure competence in basic GI flexible endoscopy.[37] FES simulator scores will be correlated with GAGES scores as part of the validation study.

Once the FES simulator has been shown to be reliable and associated with valid metrics of performance, it will then be ready to be used as an assessment tool. This stage will require describing the sensitivity and specificity of performance on the simulator by generating receiver operator curves from the simulator performance scores of physicians with varying levels of experience, as was done by Fraser and colleagues[15] for FLS. These scores will then be used to establish a cumulative score that maximizes

Date:_____

Check One: ❑ **Evaluator**   Evaluator Code: _____
                ❑ **Operator**   Operator Code: _____

GAGES - UPPER GI ENDOSCOPY SCORESHEET
GLOBAL ASSESSMENT OF GASTROINTESTINAL ENDOSCOPIC SKILLS

INTUBATION OF THE ESOPHAGUS   SCORE ☐

Reflects patient management, understanding of anatomy and sedation
5   Able to independently (successfully) intubate esophagus without patient discomfort
4
3   Requires detailed prompting and cues
2
1   Unable to properly intubate requiring take over

SCOPE NAVIGATION   SCORE ☐

Reflects navigation of the GI tract using tip deflection, advancement/withdrawal and torque
5   Expertly able to manipulated the scope in the upper GI tract autonomously.
4
3   Requires verbal guidance to completely navigate the upper GI tract
2
1   Not able to achieve goals despite detailed verbal cues, requiring take over

ABILITY TO KEEP A CLEAR ENDOSCOPIC FIELD   SCORE ☐

Utilization of insufflation, suction and/or irrigation to maximize mucosal evaluation
5   Uses insufflation, suction, and irrigation optimally to maintain clear view of endoscopic field
4
3   Requires moderate prompting to maintain clear view
2
1   Inability to maintain view despite extensive verbal cues

INSTRUMENTATION (if applicable; leave blank if not applicable) SCORE ☐

Random biopsy: targeting is assessed by asking the endoscopist to take another biopsy from the identical
site. Targeted instrumentation: evaluation is based on ability to direct the instrument to the target.
5   Expertly directs instrument to desired target
4
3   Requires some guidance and/or multiple attempts to direct instrument to target
2
1   Unable to direct instrument to target despite coaching

QUALITY OF EXAMINATION   SCORE ☐

Reflects attention to patient comfort, efficiency, and completeness of mucosal evaluation
5   Expertly completes the exam efficiently and comfortably
4
3   Requires moderate assistance to accomplish a complete and comfortable exam
2
1   Could not perform a satisfactory exam despite verbal and manual assistance requiring takeover of the procedure

OVERALL SCORE:

Fig. 15. GAGES-Upper Endoscopy, for evaluation of technical skills during clinical upper endoscopy.

the sensitivity, specificity, and positive and negative predictive values of the FES score. From this cumulative score, a pass/fail level can be determined.

FES AND FUTURE WORK

FES will be launched at the SAGES national meeting in the spring of 2010. It will be the first validated program for the teaching and evaluation of flexible GI endoscopy. It will represent 5 years of concentrated work by SAGES members to take the program from concept to reality. In the surgical world, the release of FES is much anticipated. Like

Date:_____

Check One: ❑ **Evaluator**   Evaluator Code: _____
                ❑ **Operator**   Operator Code: _____

GAGES - COLONOSCOPY SCORESHEET
GLOBAL ASSESSMENT OF GASTROINTESTINAL ENDOSCOPIC SKILLS

SCOPE NAVIGATION   SCORE ❑
Reflects navigation of the GI tract using tip deflection, advancement/withdrawal and torque
5   Expertly able to manipulate the scope in the GI tract autonomously
4
3   Requires verbal guidance to completely navigate the lower GI tract
2
1   Not able to achieve goals despite detailed verbal guidance requiring takeover

USE OF STRATEGIES   SCORE ❑
Examines use of patient positions, abdominal pressure, insufflation, suction and loop reduction to comfortably compete the procedure
5   Expert use of appropriate strategies for advancement of the scope while optimizing patient comfort
4
3   Use of some strategies appropriately, but requires moderate verbal guidance
2
1   Unable to utilize appropriate strategies for scope advancement despite verbal assistance

ABILITY TO KEEP A CLEAR ENDOSCOPIC FIELD   SCORE ❑
Utilization of insufflation, suction and/or irrigation to maximize mucosal evaluation
5   Used insufflation, suction, and irrigation optimally to maintain clear view of endoscopic field
4
3   Requires moderate prompting to maintain clear view
2
1   Inability to maintain view despite extensive verbal cues

INSTRUMENTATION (if applicable; leave blank if not applicable)   SCORE ❑
Random biopsy: targeting is assessed by asking the endoscopist to take another biopsy from the identical
site. Targeted instrumentation: evaluation is based on ability to direct the instrument to the target.
5   Expertly directs instrument to desired target
4
3   Requires some guidance and/or multiple attempts to direct instrument to target
2
1   Unable to direct instrument to target despite coaching

QUALITY OF EXAMINATION   SCORE ❑
Reflects attention to patient comfort, efficiency, and completeness of mucosal evaluation
5   Expertly completes the exam efficiently and comfortably
4
3   Requires moderate assistance to accomplish a complete and comfortable exam
2
1   Could not perform a satisfactory exam despite verbal and manual assistance requiring takeover of the procedure

OVERALL SCORE:

Fig. 16. GAGES-Colonoscopy, for evaluation of technical skills during clinical colonoscopy.

FLS, it is expected that passing FES will become a requirement to be eligible to apply to the ABS and will provide surgical training programs with a valid benchmark of performance that is much more accurate than case numbers.

SUMMARY

The concept that merits reiteration is the notion that passing FLS, and eventually FES, does not indicate that an individual is a competent surgeon or endoscopist, but that they have shown competence in the basic knowledge and technical skills required to safely perform these procedures. Just as a trainee would be expected to learn the differences between needle drivers and suture materials and how to suture and tie knots outside of the operating room, these programs attempt to ensure a basic level of knowledge and skill. Once this foundation has been established, and the skills become more natural and perhaps even automated, this frees cognitive space for the trainee to learn the anatomy, judgment, and subtleties of surgical decision making that are difficult to acquire in a simulated environment. Overall, the goal is to optimize patient safety and the use of operating-room resources, while improving the efficiency and quality of surgical education.

REFERENCES

1. Clarke JR. Making surgery safer. J Am Coll Surg 2005;200:229.
2. Strasberg SM, Hertl M, Soper NJ. An analysis of the problem of biliary injury during laparoscopic cholecystectomy. J Am Coll Surg 1995;180:101.
3. Brydges R, Farhat WA, El-Hout Y, et al. Pediatric urology training: performance-based assessment using the Fundamentals of Laparoscopic Surgery. J Surg Res 2009. [Epub ahead of print].
4. Dauster B, Steinberg AP, Vassiliou MC, et al. Validity of the MISTELS simulator for laparoscopy training in urology. J Endourol 2005;19:541.
5. Zheng B, Hur HC, Johnson S, et al. Validity of using Fundamentals of Laparoscopic Surgery (FLS) program to assess laparoscopic competence for gynecologists. Surg Endosc 2010;24(1):152–60.
6. Scott DJ, Dunnington GL. The new ACS/APDS Skills Curriculum: moving the learning curve out of the operating room. J Gastrointest Surg 2008;12:213.
7. Ritter EM, Scott DJ. Design of a proficiency-based skills training curriculum for the Fundamentals of Laparoscopic Surgery. Surg Innov 2007;14:107.
8. Scott DJ, Ritter EM, Tesfay ST, et al. Certification pass rate of 100% for Fundamentals of Laparoscopic Surgery skills after proficiency-based training. Surg Endosc 2008;22:1887.
9. Stefanidis D, Korndorffer JR Jr, Heniford BT, et al. Limited feedback and video tutorials optimize learning and resource utilization during laparoscopic simulator training. Surgery 2007;142:202.
10. Derossis AM, Antoniuk M, Fried GM. Evaluation of laparoscopic skills: a 2-year follow-up during residency training. Can J Surg 1999;42:293.
11. Vassiliou MC, Ghitulescu GA, Feldman LS, et al. The MISTELS program to measure technical skill in laparoscopic surgery: evidence for reliability. Surg Endosc 2006;20:744.
12. Peters JH, Fried GM, Swanstrom LL, et al. Development and validation of a comprehensive program of education and assessment of the basic Fundamentals of Laparoscopic Surgery. Surgery 2004;135:21.
13. Fried GM, Feldman LS, Vassiliou MC, et al. Proving the value of simulation in laparoscopic surgery. Ann Surg 2004;240:518.
14. Swanstrom LL, Fried GM, Hoffman KI, et al. Beta test results of a new system assessing competence in laparoscopic surgery. J Am Coll Surg 2006;202:62.
15. Fraser SA, Klassen DR, Feldman LS, et al. Evaluating laparoscopic skills: setting the pass/fail score for the MISTELS system. Surg Endosc 2003;17:964.
16. Feldman LS, Hagarty SE, Ghitulescu G, et al. Relationship between objective assessment of technical skills and subjective in-training evaluations in surgical residents. J Am Coll Surg 2004;198:105.
17. Fried GM, Derossis AM, Bothwell J, et al. Comparison of laparoscopic performance in vivo with performance measured in a laparoscopic simulator. Surg Endosc 1999;13:1077.

18. Vassiliou MC, Feldman LS, Andrew CG, et al. A global assessment tool for evaluation of intraoperative laparoscopic skills. Am J Surg 2005;190:107.
19. McCluney AL, Vassiliou MC, Kaneva PA, et al. FLS simulator performance predicts intraoperative laparoscopic skill. Surg Endosc 2007;21:1991.
20. Feldman LS, Cao J, Andalib A, et al. A method to characterize the learning curve for performance of a fundamental laparoscopic simulator task: defining "learning plateau" and "learning rate". Surgery 2009;146:381.
21. Fraser SA, Feldman LS, Stanbridge D, et al. Characterizing the learning curve for a basic laparoscopic drill. Surg Endosc 2005;19:1572.
22. Castellvi AO, Hollett LA, Minhajuddin A, et al. Maintaining proficiency after Fundamentals of Laparoscopic Surgery training: a 1-year analysis of skill retention for surgery residents. Surgery 2009;146:387.
23. Stefanidis D, Acker C, Heniford BT. Proficiency-based laparoscopic simulator training leads to improved operating room skill that is resistant to decay. Surg Innov 2008;15:69.
24. Stefanidis D, Korndorffer JR Jr, Markley S, et al. Proficiency maintenance: impact of ongoing simulator training on laparoscopic skill retention. J Am Coll Surg 2006; 202:599.
25. Stefanidis D, Walters KC, Mostafavi A, et al. What is the ideal interval between training sessions during proficiency-based laparoscopic simulator training? Am J Surg 2009;197:126.
26. Hsu KE, Man FY, Gizicki RA, et al. Experienced surgeons can do more than one thing at a time: effect of distraction on performance of a simple laparoscopic and cognitive task by experienced and novice surgeons. Surg Endosc 2008;22:196.
27. Zheng B, Cassera MA, Martinec DV, et al. Measuring mental workload during the performance of advanced laparoscopic tasks. Surg Endosc 2010;24(1):45–50.
28. Sroka G, Feldman LS, Vassiliou MC, et al. Fundamentals of Laparoscopic Surgery simulator training to proficiency improves laparoscopic performance in the operating room—a randomized controlled trial. Am J Surg 2010;199(1):115–20.
29. Okrainec A, Smith L, Azzie G. Surgical simulation in Africa: the feasibility and impact of a 3-day Fundamentals of Laparoscopic Surgery course. Surg Endosc 2009. [Epub ahead of print].
30. Okrainec A, Henao O, Azzie G. Telesimulation: an effective method for teaching the Fundamentals of Laparoscopic Surgery in resource-restricted countries. Surg Endosc 2010;24(2):417–22.
31. Soper NJ, Fried GM. The Fundamentals of Laparoscopic Surgery: its time has come. Bull Am Coll Surg 2008;93:30.
32. Derevianko AY, Schwaitzberg SD, Tsuda S, et al. Malpractice carrier underwrites Fundamentals of Laparoscopic Surgery training and testing: a benchmark for patient safety. Surg Endosc 2010;24(3):616–23.
33. Bittner JG 4th, Marks JM, Dunkin B, et al. Resident training in flexible gastrointestinal endoscopy: a review of current issues and options. J Surg Educ 2007;64:399.
34. Cass OW. Objective evaluation of competence: technical skills in gastrointestinal endoscopy. Endoscopy 1995;27:86.
35. Reed WP, Kilkenny JW, Dias CE, et al. A prospective analysis of 3525 esophagogastroduodenoscopies performed by surgeons. Surg Endosc 2004;18:11.
36. Wexner SD, Garbus JE, Singh JJ. A prospective analysis of 13,580 colonoscopies. Reevaluation of credentialing guidelines. Surg Endosc 2001;15:251.
37. Vassiliou MC, Kaneva P, Poulose BK, et al. GAGES: A valid measurement tool for technical skills in flexible endoscopy. Surg Endosc 2010. [Epub ahead of print].

Verification of Proficiency: A Prerequisite for Clinical Experience

Hilary Sanfey, MB, BCh, Gary Dunnington, MD*

KEYWORDS
- Surgical skills training • Surgery • Proficiency

For more than a century, residents received their technical training exclusively in the operating room, and performed procedures based on patient availability without attention to individual learner needs. More recently, several factors have led to the introduction of dedicated skills laboratories and a more widespread belief in the value of time spent in skills training.[1–8] The impetus for change in our approach to teaching technical skills has been driven by a reduction in resident work hours, concerns about patient safety, and the challenge of achieving technical proficiency with emerging technology. The educational rationale for skills training in a laboratory setting is based on established theories of learning in which the trainee passes through cognitive, integrative, and autonomous stages of learning.[9] Deliberate practice is one of the fundamental elements proven to encourage automaticity and improve motor-skill abilities. Deliberative practice requires that the learners repeatedly perform well-defined, level-appropriate tasks, and receive immediate feedback that allows for correction of errors.[9–12] Therefore, the earlier stages of teaching technical skills should take place outside the operating room to permit deliberative practice and allow the trainee to focus on more complex patient care and management issues in the clinical situation. In past models of surgical training that were based primarily on apprenticeship, these opportunities for deliberate practice were rare.

EVALUATION OF SKILLS TRAINING

Evaluation is essential to document learner performance and proficiency, provide learner feedback, and gather data for performance standards. It is therefore an important component of skills instruction. In their 2005 paper, Williams and colleagues[13] identified six major factors that compromise the process of observing, measuring,

Department of Surgery, Southern Illinois University School of Medicine, PO Box 19638, Springfield, IL 62794, USA
* Corresponding author.
E-mail address: gdunnington@siumed.edu

Surg Clin N Am 90 (2010) 559–567
doi:10.1016/j.suc.2010.02.008   surgical.theclinics.com
0039-6109/10/$ – see front matter © 2010 Elsevier Inc. All rights reserved.

and characterizing a resident performance. In order of importance, these factors are: (1) incomplete sampling of performance, (2) rater memory constraints or distortion, (3) hidden performance deficits of the resident, (4) lack of meaningful benchmarks, (5) faculty members' hesitancy to act on negative performance information, and (6) systematic rater error. The investigators offered practical solutions to overcome these problems and these are summarized in **Table 1**. These principles should guide all forms of performance assessment including the implementation of skills evaluation.

Researchers have developed several validated instruments for evaluating the technical aspects of surgical performance.[1,14–23] One such example is the Objective Structured Assessment of Technical Skills (OSATS).[19,20] The OSATS is a performance-based examination designed to assess the technical-skill competence of surgical trainees in which candidates perform a series of standardized surgical tasks under the direct observation of an expert.[17,19,20] Examiners score candidates using a task-specific checklist consisting of 10 to 30 essential elements of the procedure and a global rating form. This form includes five to eight surgical behaviors, such as respect for tissues, economy of motion, and appropriate use of assistants. An export of this evaluation to nine programs in the Chicago and Los Angeles areas demonstrated psychometric properties that are highly consistent with previously reported data suggesting that the examination is portable.[24] In one of the most comprehensive skills lab curriculum evaluations reported to date, Anastakis and colleagues[25] used the OSATS and trainee evaluations to conduct a formative evaluation of the Surgical Skills Centre Curriculum at the University of Toronto. Historical controls were compared with resident participants and results indicated that single session training on a procedure would not yield a lasting effect on a resident's performance, a finding that is supported in the expertise and motor learning literature.[25] Anastakis and colleagues emphasized the need for ongoing repetitive practice.

Table 1
Factors that compromise the process of measuring resident performance and suggested solutions

Problem	Solution
Inadequate sampling	Maximize number of ratings and sample broadly Observe all aspects of a performance
Memory distortion	Evaluate and give immediate feedback, Encourage immediate recording Limit number of items
Hidden performance deficits caused by collective nature of work	Performance examinations Observe a wide range of activities
Lack of meaningful benchmarks	Resist changing the form to follow trends Develop rating norms Carry out longitudinal analysis
Hesitancy to act	Seek performance reports only Do not ask faculty to assign grade or make promotion recommendation Make progress decisions by committee
Systematic rater error	Increase number of raters Familiarize raters with evaluation form

Data from Williams R, Dunnington G, Klamen D, et al. Forecasting residents' performance – partly cloudy. Acad Med 2005;80(5):415–22.

Other methods of assessment in the laboratory setting include the McGill Inanimate System for Training and Evaluation of Laparoscopic Skills (MISTELS)[26] and the Imperial College Surgical Assessment Device (ICSAD).[15,27] Developed at McGill University in Montreal, the MISTELS uses an inanimate box to simulate the generic skills needed in the performance of laparoscopic surgery. It is a valid and reliable instrument for assessing laparoscopic skills.[26] The ICSAD, developed at Imperial College in London, tracks hand motion using sensors placed on the trainee's hands during the performance of a task. The sensors translate movement into a computerized tracing of hand motion, which provides an effective index of technical skill in laparoscopic[27] and open procedures.[15,28] This index has good concordance with OSATS scores.

VERIFICATION OF PROFICIENCY

The American College of Surgeons (ACS) and the Association of Program Directors in Surgery (APDS) have established a three-phase skills curriculum for all surgery residents.[29] Phase 1 involves basic surgical skills instructional modules and a Verification of Proficiency (VOP) assessment. Proficiency-based training refers to the concept of learners practicing certain surgical skills until testing shows them to be at a predetermined target level of ability. Ahlberg and colleagues[30] demonstrated that such training by novices on a virtual reality simulator leads to fewer errors during operating room performance than for those learners who did not experience proficiency-based training. Stefanidis and colleagues[31] showed that training novices to proficiency using basic laparoscopic models translated to improved performance on live-animal models, which was durable over a period of months. The Verification of Proficiency assessment tool, developed at Southern Illinois University (SIU), was selected by the curriculum design team as a more faculty friendly alternative to the OSATs for assessment of the basic skills included in Phase 1 of the curriculum.

Since 2005, the Department of Surgery at SIU has employed the ACS/APDS basic surgical skills curriculum in its training laboratory for first-year surgical residents (PGY1 residents). The goal is to provide these trainees with a foundation of motor skills and background knowledge for further learning in the operating room. Using this curriculum, matriculating PGY1 residents can be trained to the technical ability of mid-level surgical residents in multiple skills and procedures within a period of weeks.[32] The authors have developed several VOP modules for teaching and evaluating basic surgical skills. Each module includes objectives for performance, guidelines for practice, and instructions for VOP testing. These modules are listed in **Table 2**. All PGY1 residents from general surgery and the four surgical specialty programs (orthopedic surgery, otolaryngology, plastic surgery, and urology) undergo VOP evaluation on the basic surgical skills (see **Table 2**) at the beginning of their first year of surgical residency. Instruction and VOP evaluation on the procedural skills (see **Table 2**) takes place later in the first year and early in the second year to coincide with performance of these procedures on clinical rotations. Residents view a video of an expert performance followed by a period of faculty-led instruction and guided practice. Residents are tested on each module after a period of learner-determined practice with a skills coach. Performances are videotaped with the Medical Education Technologies Inc (METI) Learning automated video capturing system (**Fig. 1**).[33] The METI Learning system allows raters to annotate resident errors on the video for specific learner feedback at a later date. De-identified videos are scored by surgical faculty on the system's Web-based interface from their office or other remote computers, using the ACS/APDS VOP rating forms. Kopta[34] reported high inter-rater reliability using checklists to assess surgical skills, and later studies by Regehr and others

Table 2
Verification of proficiency modules in use at Southern Illinois University School of Medicine

Basic Surgical Skills	Procedural Skills
Knot tying (5 modules)	Esophagogastroduodenoscopy
Basic suturing (3 modules)	Colonoscopy
Central venous access	Biopsy
Chest tube placement	Arterial anastomosis
Emergency surgical airway	Bowel anastomosis
	Basic laparoscopic skills
	Laparoscopic cholecystectomy

demonstrated that global ratings are better able to differentiate the abilities of junior versus senior residents.[35] Therefore, the authors have incorporated a checklist of specific performance characteristics for feedback purposes and an overall final global rating, stating whether the individual demonstrates proficiency or requires additional practice, into the VOP rating forms. Residents scored as needing additional practice on this final rating are deemed to have failed that VOP and undergo a period of mandatory remediation. An example of one of the proficiency evaluation forms is demonstrated in **Fig. 2**.The procedural modules also include a rating of economy of time and motion and space for evaluator comments and feedback. These evaluation instruments, in addition to their utility in the verification of proficiency process, also allow for feedback about specific aspects of the performance. The VOP method of evaluation has a considerable advantage over OSATS in that evaluation by direct observation

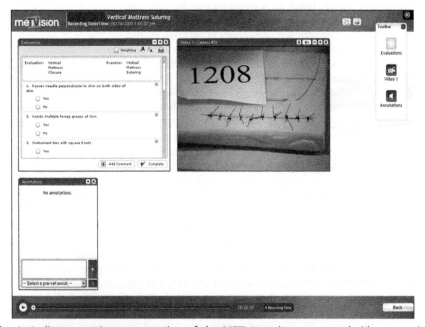

Fig. 1. A diagrammatic representation of the METI Learning automated video capturing system in use at SIU. The rater has the ability to simultaneously view the performance on video and rate it on the VOP rating form. Performance deficits can be annotated to provide specific feedback to the learner.

| SUBCUTICULAR SKIN CLOSURE | Resident: _____ | | Date: _____ |

SKIN SUTURING STEPS	Yes	No
Runs the suture, placing appropriate bites into dermal layer		
Enters the dermal layer directly across from exit site		
Avoids penetration of the epidermis		
Avoids multiple forcep grasps of skin		
Instrument ties with square knots		
Approximates skin with appropriate tension		

1	2	3	4	5
Economy of Time and Motion	Many unnecessary / disorganized movements	Organized time / motion, some unnecessary movement		Maximum economy of movement and efficiency

Final Rating	Other Summative Comments:
❏ Demonstrates competence	
❏ Requires further practice	Evaluator _____

Fig. 2. An example of one of the Verification Evaluation Forms in use at SIU. All forms have a procedure-specific checklist and a global rating item.

does not have to take place at the time of testing but can occur at any time and place convenient to the faculty rater. Over the past two years, 65% of residents failed at least one module and 48% failed at least two modules at the first attempt. Residents who failed underwent a period of remediation and were subsequently retested until deemed proficient on each module.

At SIU, residents are required to demonstrate proficiency on each of the procedural modules before performing that procedure under supervision in the operating room. For example, trainees must demonstrate proficiency in the performance of a laparoscopic cholecystectomy in a porcine model before performing that operation on patients. As a method of formative evaluation, VOP provides a framework to determine individual learner progress toward proficiency in the skills laboratory. As high-stakes assessment, VOP seeks to ensure that novice trainees have the basic technical skills necessary to be safe participants in actual clinical procedures; those residents who do not pass particular VOP evaluations are not allowed to function as the primary operating surgeon in the corresponding procedures in the operating room. A preliminary analysis of some of the VOP instrument properties have been reported as part of an earlier study.[32] Selected instruments have the ability to discriminate between untrained novices and those who have undergone the training curriculum for four different surgical skills. In addition, the inter-rater agreement on these evaluations was excellent (>0.87).[32] Work is continuing to study and refine the beta versions of the Phase 1 VOP instruments, as a first step toward developing a national proficiency examination for basic surgical skills in PGY1 residents.

DISCUSSION

The literature on measurement of basic surgical skills has primarily focused on assessment in the laboratory setting, but more recently has begun to investigate transfer of that ability to clinical practice.[19,36] In addition to using measurement of skills for formative assessment, there has been some initial work on setting passing standards for skills assessments.[37–40] Even more recent has been the movement toward proficiency-based training in skills laboratories for the purpose of improved performance in the operating room. To date, the evidence for transfer to the operating room is stronger for minimally invasive surgery than for open procedures. In a series of experiments involving more than 200 surgeons and trainees, practice on a laparoscopic simulator led to the acquisition of skills that were transferable to complex laparoscopic tasks, such as suturing.[26] Similarly, second- and third-year residents who received formal training on a laparoscopic simulator had a significantly greater improvement in video-trainer scores and global assessments of performance of a laparoscopic cholecystectomy compared with residents who had no simulator training.[41] The transfer of skills learned on virtual reality laparoscopic simulators has also been encouraging. Residents who received virtual reality training performed the dissection more quickly, made fewer errors, and had higher economy-of-movement scores during a laparoscopic cholecystectomy than did residents without such training.[39,42] Taken together, these studies strongly suggest that ex vivo laparoscopic training leads to detectable benefits for learners in clinical settings, although it is unclear whether the improvement in performance after ex vivo training is durable.[43,44] Nonetheless, one could argue that although the advantages of training on a simulator may be limited to early procedural experience, the enhanced early learning curve may allow educators to be more efficient with their time. Finally, there are data to suggest that high fidelity may be less important at junior levels of training.[45,46]

SUMMARY

Surgical educators need to incorporate meaningful assessment into residency programs, using rigorous, reliable, and regular means of testing for surgical skills. For example, the VOP could be used to assess a resident's performance on basic surgical skills and the MISTELS program might be used to assess a resident's performance of basic laparoscopic skills. Similarly, either OSATS stations or the operative performance rating system could be used to assess performance during open procedures. Residents would thus be trained in the laboratory until preset criteria had been met and would only then be allowed to participate in the performance of procedures in patients. Competence-based advancement, rather than time served, would become the standard in surgical training.

Although many research studies have described systems of assessment of surgical skills, there is no clear estimate of the extent to which surgical programs are using any sort of assessment in their skills laboratories. Previous surveys have established consensus opinions on the educational value of skills laboratory curricula, but have not identified how skills' testing is incorporated into residency curricula or how it might be used for decisions about resident advancement or matriculation.[47,48] Currently, the only measure of satisfactory completion of operative training is number of cases performed[49] and end-of-rotation ratings by attending surgeons. Both have limitations; the operative log simply indicates the frequency of procedures performed without regard to quality of the process or outcomes, and end-of-rotation ratings provide a generalized evaluation of resident performance rather than evaluations of specific operative procedures. In addition, the timing of completion of these evaluations is subject to rating errors caused by selective recall and time delay in completion. The ability to videotape a performance and review and evaluate it at leisure will significantly reduce these errors and improve the reliability of performance evaluation.

One of the challenges of a competence-based system of education and assessment that has received little attention is how to establish pass or fail standards for the performance of technical skills. This is a major deficit in the assessment literature that will require attention if a criterion-based system is implemented or if certification of technical ability is required before licensure. One of the opportunities provided by the ACS/APDS National Curriculum is the possibility to perform multi-institutional studies that will allow us to gather data to improve the assessment and training of surgeons in the future. Work is continuing to study and refine the beta versions of the Phase 1 VOP instruments as a first step toward developing a national proficiency examination for basic surgical skills in PGY1 residents.

REFERENCES

1. Cauraugh JH, Martin M, Martin KK. Modeling surgical expertise for motor skill acquisition. Am J Surg 1999;177:331–6.
2. Hamstra SJ, Dubrowski A. Effective training and assessment of surgical skills, and the correlates of performance. Surg Innov 2005;12:71–7.
3. Heppell J, Beauchamp G, Chollet A. Ten-year experience with a basic technical skills and perioperative management workshop for first-year residents. Can J Surg 1995;38:27–32.
4. Hutchison C, Hamstra S, Leadbetter W. The University of Toronto Surgical Skills Centre opens. Focus Surg Educ 1998;16:22–4.
5. Lossing AG, Hatswell EM, Gilas T, et al. A technical-skills course for 1st-year residents in general surgery: a descriptive study. Can J Surg 1992;35:536–40.
6. Reznick RK. Teaching and testing technical skills. Am J Surg 1993;165:358–61.
7. Reznick RK, MacRae H. Teaching surgical skills — changes in the wind. N Engl J Med 2006;355(25):2664–9.
8. Scallon SE, Fairholm DJ, Cochrane DD, et al. Evaluation of the operating room as a surgical teaching venue. Can J Surg 1992;35:173–6.
9. Fitts PM, Posner MI. Human performance. Belmont (CA): Brooks/Cole; 1967.
10. Ericsson KA. The acquisition of expert performance: an introduction to some of the issues. In: Ericsson KA, editor. The road to excellence: the acquisition of expert performance in the arts and sciences, sports, and games. Mahwah (NJ): Lawrence Erlbaum Associates; 1996. p. 1–50.
11. Ericsson KA. Deliberate practice and the acquisition and maintenance of expert performance in medicine and related domains. Acad Med 2004;79(Suppl 10):S70–81.
12. Ericsson K, Krampe R, Tesch-Romer C. The role of deliberate practice in the acquisition of expert performance. Psychol Rev 1993;100:363–406.
13. Williams R, Dunnington G, Klamen D, et al. Forecasting residents' performance – partly cloudy. Acad Med 2005;80(5):415–22.
14. Aggarwal R, Grantcharov T, Moorthy K, et al. An evaluation of the feasibility, validity and reliability of laparoscopic skills assessment in the operating room. Ann Surg 2007;245(6):992–9.
15. Datta V, Mackay SD, Mandalia M, et al. The use of electromagnetic motion tracking analysis to objectively measure open surgical skill in the laboratory-based model. J Am Coll Surg 2001;193:479–85.
16. Dunnington G, DaRosa D, Kolm P. Development of a model for evaluating teaching in the operating room. Curr Surg 1993;50:523–7.
17. Faulkner H, Regehr G, Martin J, et al. Validation of an objective structured assessment of technical skill for surgical residents. Acad Med 1996;71:1363–5.
18. Mackay S, Datta V, Chang A, et al. Multiple objective measures of skills (MOMS): a new approach to the assessment of technical ability in surgical trainees. Ann Surg 2003;238(2):291–300.

19. Martin JA, Regehr G, Reznick R, et al. Objective Structured Assessment of Technical Skill (OSATS) for surgical residents. Br J Surg 1997;84:273–8.
20. Reznick R, Regehr G, MacRae H, et al. Testing technical skill via an innovative "bench station" examination. Am J Surg 1997;173:226–30.
21. Tang B, Hanna GB, Carter F, et al. Competence assessment of laparoscopic operative and cognitive skills: objective structured clinical examination (OSCE) or observational clinical human reliability assessment (OCHRA). World J Surg 2006;30(4):527–34.
22. Vassilou M, Feldman LS, Andrew CG, et al. A global assessment tool for evaluation of intraoperative laparoscopic skills. Am J Surg 2005;190(1):107–13.
23. Yule S, Flin R, Paterson-Brown S, et al. Developing a taxonomy of surgeon's non – technical skills. Med Educ 2006;40:1098–104.
24. Ault G, Reznick R, MacRae H, et al. Exporting a technical skills evaluation technology to other sites. Am J Surg 2001;182(3):254–6.
25. Anastakis DJ, Wanzel KR, Brown MH, et al. Evaluating the effectiveness of a 2-year curriculum in a surgical skills center. Am J Surg 2003;185:378–85.
26. Fried GM, Feldman LS, Vassiliou MC, et al. Proving the value of simulation in laparoscopic surgery. Ann Surg 2004;240:518–28.
27. Taffinder N, Sutton C, Fishwick RJ, et al. Validation of virtual reality to teach and assess psychomotor skills in laparoscopic surgery: results from randomised controlled studies using the MIST VR laparoscopic simulator. Stud Health Technol Inform 1998;50:124–30.
28. Darzi A, Mackay S. Assessment of surgical competence. Qual Health Care 2001; 10(Suppl 2):ii64–9.
29. ACS/APDS. Surgical skills curriculum information. American College of Surgeons: Division of Education; 2008. Available at: http://elearning.facs.org/course/view.php?id=3. Accessed October 22, 2009.
30. Ahlberg G, Enochsson L, Gallagher AG, et al. Proficiency-based virtual reality training significantly reduces the error rate for residents during their first 10 laparoscopic cholecystectomies. Am J Surg 2007;193(6):797–804.
31. Stefanidis D, Acker C, Heniford BT. Proficiency-based laparoscopic simulator training leads to improved operating room skill that is resistant to decay. Surg Innov 2008;15(1):69–73.
32. Boehler ML, Schwind CJ, Rogers DA, et al. A theory-based curriculum for enhancing surgical skillfulness. J Am Coll Surg 2007;205(3):492–7.
33. METI learning. Available at: http://www.meti.com/main_faq.htm. Accessed October 24, 2009.
34. Kopta JA. An approach to evaluation of operative skills. Surgery 1971;70: 297–303.
35. Regehr G, MacRae H, Reznick RK, et al. Comparing the psychometric properties of checklists and global rating scales for assessing performance on an OSCE-format examination. Acad Med 1998;73:993–7.
36. Park J, MacRae H, Musselman LJ, et al. Randomized controlled trial of virtual reality simulator training: transfer to live patients. Am J Surg 2007;194(2):205–11.
37. Fraser SA, Klassen DR, Feldman LS, et al. Evaluating laparoscopic skills: setting the pass/fail score for the MISTELS system. Surg Endosc 2003;17(6):964–7.
38. Grantcharov TP, Kristiansen VB, Bendix J, et al. Randomized clinical trial of virtual reality simulation for laparoscopic skills training. Br J Surg 2004;91:146–50.
39. Grantcharov TP, Schulze S, Kristiansen VB. The impact of objective assessment and constructive feedback on improvement of laparoscopic performance in the operating room. Surg Endosc 2007;21(12):2240–3.

40. Hauge LS. Evaluating the skills lab curriculum and instruction. In: ACS/APDS, editor. Surgical skills curriculum information. American College of Surgeons: Division of Education; 2008. Available at: http://elearning.facs.org/course/view.php?id=3. Accessed October 10, 2009.
41. Scott DJ, Bergen PC, Rege RV, et al. Laparoscopic training on bench models: better and more cost effective than operating room experience? J Am Coll Surg 2000;191:272–83.
42. Seymour NE, Gallagher AG, Roman SA, et al. Virtual reality training improves operating room performance: results of a randomized, double-blinded study. Ann Surg 2002;236:458–63.
43. Grober ED, Hamstra SJ, Wanzel KR, et al. Laboratory based training in urologic microsurgery with bench model simulators: a randomized controlled trial evaluating the durability of technical skill. J Urol 2004;172:378–81.
44. Sedlack RE, Kolars JC. Computer simulator training enhances the competency of gastroenterology fellows at colonoscopy: results of a pilot study. Am J Gastroenterol 2004;99(1):33–7.
45. Matsumoto ED, Hamstra SJ, Radomski SB, et al. The effect of bench model fidelity on endourological skills: a randomized controlled study. J Urol 2002; 167:1243–7.
46. Anastakis DJ, Regehr G, Reznick RK, et al. Assessment of technical skills transfer from the bench training model to the human model. Am J Surg 1999;177:167–70.
47. Kapadia MR, DaRosa DA, MacRae HM, et al. Current assessment and future directions of surgical skills laboratories. J Surg Educ 2007;64(5):260–5.
48. Korndorffer JR Jr, Stefanidis D, Scott DJ. Laparoscopic skills laboratories: current assessment and a call for resident training standards. Am J Surg 2006;191(1): 17–22.
49. Haluck RS, Krummel TM. Computers and virtual reality for surgical education in the 21st century. Arch Surg 2000;135:786–92.

Surgical Team Training: Promoting High Reliability with Nontechnical Skills

John T. Paige, MD

KEYWORDS

- Team training • High reliability • Nontechnical skills
- Operating room • Teamwork

The past decade has witnessed an ongoing transformation in surgical training in the United States and abroad, led in large part by the incorporation of simulation into residency educational curricula. As a result, the Halstedian apprentice-based teaching model, founded on the maxim of "See one, do one, teach one," is steadily giving way to an objectives-based educational model centered around the triad of targeted task performance, immediate feedback, and repeated focused practice associated with Ericsson's conceptual framework of deliberate practice.[1] This paradigm shift in *how* surgery is taught has also been accompanied by an expansion in *what* is taught, as surgical educators have realized the importance of organization- and team-based dynamics in the care of the surgical patient. To succeed in today's health care environment, a surgeon must be more than a masterful technician; he or she must be an expert team leader with a firm grasp of how the system in which he or she operates functions.

This article focuses on key aspects of these "nontraditional" surgical subjects of organizational structure and team interaction. First, the deficiencies in team dynamics found within the modern operating room (OR) and their resultant consequences are highlighted. Next, essential human factors concepts related to error generation, organizational culture, high reliability, and team science as applied to the OR environment are reviewed. Finally, various strategies for improving OR team function, including the use of high-fidelity simulation (HFS) in team training are discussed.

MODERN OPERATING ROOM TEAM DYNAMICS AND THEIR CONSEQUENCES

The modern OR is a highly dynamic work environment that brings together a diverse group of professionals who must work effectively together as a team to provide safe,

Department of Surgery, Louisiana State University School of Medicine, 1542 Tulane Avenue, Room 734, New Orleans, LA 70112, USA
E-mail address: jpaige@lsuhsc.edu

Surg Clin N Am 90 (2010) 569–581
doi:10.1016/j.suc.2010.02.007   surgical.theclinics.com
0039-6109/10/$ – see front matter © 2010 Elsevier Inc. All rights reserved.

quality care to the surgical patient. In such a high-risk environment, each team member must draw upon his or her expert clinical knowledge as well as several distinct categories of skills (**Table 1**).[2,3] Nontechnical skills (NTS) are the combination of those cognitive and interpersonal skills that complement each team member's technical skills to contribute to a safe, effective operative intervention.[2,4] They form the foundation on which team interaction and dynamics are built. Fortunately, NTS are not innately derived; instead, they can be acquired through teaching and training, much like technical skills are learned.[5]

That NTS are teachable skills is encouraging, especially given the dysfunctional status of current OR team dynamics. Indeed, the modern OR team is more appropriately characterized as a group of experts rather than an expert team.[6] Members favor *multi*professional practice over *inter*professional collaboration.[7] The resultant "silo mentality" that each profession brings to the OR is reinforced only by its ready stereotyping of the "other" professions working on the OR team.[8] Finally, differentials in both status and the frequency of individual traits such as motivation, competitiveness, and dominance among the various OR professions contribute to a hierarchical structure prone to interprofessional friction.[9]

This multiprofessional nature of practice within the modern OR allows each profession to harbor divergent conceptions of appropriate team interactions and norms. For example, McDonald and colleagues[10] demonstrated that nurses' reliance on adherence to written rules of conduct and standardized approaches to therapy were in direct conflict with surgeons' beliefs in following unwritten rules of established behavior and maintaining flexibility in treatment plans. These differing attitudes related to behavior and clinical decision making negatively affected trust between the two professions. Additionally, Undre and colleagues[11] revealed that the definition of the term "team" itself differed among OR professions. Whereas nurses tended to view an "OR team" as a unit made up of members working together, surgeons and anesthesiologists took the more traditional view of the "OR team" as a grouping of specialists working within defined boundaries (ie, silos).

The divergent conceptions of team combine with stereotyping to distort each profession's perception of each other and their performance in the OR. Lingard and colleagues[12] found that each profession's self-described role on the OR team was in fact discordant with how other professions within the OR viewed that profession's

Table 1
Operating room skill categories

Category	Example
Technical skills	Endotracheal intubation Patient positioning Suturing
Cognitive skills	Decision making Planning Analytical thinking
Interpersonal skills	Communication Assertiveness Conflict resolution

Data from Fletcher GCL, McGeorge P, Flin RH, et al. The role of non-technical skills in anesthesia: a review of current literature. Br J Anaesth 2002;88:418–429; North Carolina State University Counseling Center. Interpersonal skills. Available at: http://www.ncsu.edu/counseling_center/resources/personal/interpersonal_skills/interpersonal_skills.htm. Accessed October 31, 2009.

responsibilities. Flin and colleagues[13] showed that this disconnect extended to perceived leadership style. Whereas most surgeons described their leadership as consultative, a similar proportion of nurses viewed it as autocratic. Moorthy and colleagues[14] and Paige and colleagues[15] revealed a tendency for a profession to overestimate its self-assessed contribution to team function compared with observer- or peer-based ratings. Finally, Makary and colleagues[16] demonstrated marked differences among the professions in each one's perception of the quality of teamwork within the OR. For example, surgeons perceived teamwork with nurses within the OR as good at an almost twofold higher rate than nurses' views of the same interaction.

Communication suffers in the OR multiprofessional practice model as well. Lingard and colleagues[17] discovered that up to one-third of all communications within the OR fail in their purpose. The reasons for these breakdowns are manifold, ranging from poor timing of the communication to exclusion of key team members from the communication. Such ineffective communication naturally can lead to increased tension within the OR.[18] Finally, the poor communication is likely magnified by an OR culture that discourages members from alerting each other regarding potential threats within the environment[19] and the poor interpersonal skills of other members on the OR team.[20]

The silo mentality, divergent perceptions of team-based roles and performance, and poor communication among the professions within the modern OR negatively affect team function as well as surgical patient care. Rosenstein and O'Daniel[21] discovered that disruptive behavior such as yelling and the use of abusive language is unfortunately commonplace, increasing frustration and stress within the OR. More telling, it further stifles communication and interprofessional collaboration, leading many OR team members to link such behavior with decreased patient safety and quality of care. Christian and colleagues[22] established an even stronger link between team dysfunction and quality of care by revealing that difficulties with workload distribution and communication in complex surgical cases have the potential of negatively affecting patient safety. Finally, Mishra and colleagues[23] linked breakdowns in NTS with increased rates of error in technical skills within the OR.

Most importantly, impaired team dynamics in the modern OR is responsible for both adverse events and poor outcomes. Communication breakdowns have been linked to wrong-site surgery[24,25] as well as other adverse events.[26] Mazzocco and colleagues[27] have even shown that poor teamwork in the OR results in higher postoperative morbidity (ie, complication rates) and mortality. Clearly, improving team dynamics in the OR should be a priority and has the potential to improve processes and outcomes of surgical care.

THE OPERATING ROOM TEAM FROM A HUMAN FACTORS PERSPECTIVE

Human factors, or ergonomics, is the study of the interaction of humans with their environment. As such, it strives to understand the physical and psychological factors at play when humans interface with machines, systems, or other humans to create safe work environments that maximize efficiency. A central tenet of the field is the *inevitability of error* occurring in any system designed or operated by humans because of the innate *fallibility of humans*.[28] Consequently, an understanding of the *conditions* under which humans work within a complex system is paramount for designing layers of defense, so-called *defenses-in-depth*, to trap and mitigate the impact of errors within that system.[29,30] Even so, each layer within a series of defenses-in-depth is susceptible to dynamic defects that, when they become aligned with defects within all the other layers, create a "window of opportunity" for catastrophic failure.[31] Defects typically arise from one of two sources: (1) *active failures* occurring at the "sharp-end" of the human-system interface that have immediate but short-lived impacts and (2) *latent conditions* occurring at the organizational level that lie dormant within a system until a confluence of local circumstances reveal them.[31] Within this context, the OR team can be a dual source of weakness. It can contribute to the formation of a defect within the defenses-in-depth of a system via active failure by members working at the "sharp-end" of care or as a latent condition owing to the dysfunctional nature of team dynamics.

The OR can be considered one of many clinical microsystems dedicated to a common patient care purpose that help make up the organizational structure of a health care entity.[32] As such, it operates within the cultural climate of the larger institution of which it is a part. Westrum[33] defined three main types of organizational cultures with distinct responses to failure: (1) the power-oriented pathologic culture that attempts to find scapegoats and suppress the problem; (2) the rules-oriented bureaucratic culture that focuses on meting out justice and providing local fixes; and (3) the performance-oriented generative culture that embraces failure as an opportunity for improvement and searches for its root causes. Understanding the way in which an organizational culture processes information and responds to error is critical in developing an effective approach to improving OR team dynamics within a particular health care system, especially because the best way to support cultural change is by addressing real problems in ways that will promote participation and successfully shift assumptions to tilt the organizational culture in the desired direction.[34]

A generative organizational culture is characteristic of *high-reliability organizations* (HROs). These organizations promote a *culture of safety* in which safety becomes the organization's *primary priority*.[35] Because HROs recognize as an illusion the possibility of becoming completely safe, they maintain a constant *preoccupation with failure*.[36] As a result, they pay particularly close attention to frontline operations in an effort to find weaknesses in their defenses.[37] In HROs, expertise trumps rank, safety becomes everyone's responsibility, and resilience in the face of failure allows for systems to function in times of crisis.[36,37] HROs, however, cannot exist without highly reliable teams (HRTs) functioning within them.[5] In this context, improving the function of the OR team takes on even more urgency, as HRO status is unattainable without it.

Before becoming an HRT, the multiprofessional practice of the OR must become a team. Currently, it is a working group of siloed individuals who, in the best circumstances, act as a potential team and, in the worse situations, function more like a pseudo-team.[38] By definition, teams in health care possess five key attributes: (1) they consist of two or more individuals; (2) they consist of members with specific roles and tasks who interact to achieve a common goal; (3) they have the ability to make decisions; (4) they have specialized knowledge and skill for use in a high workload environment; and (5) they have collective action arising from task interdependency.[39]

According to LePine and colleagues,[40] team actions and activities can be divided into three specific second-order processes that are themselves governed by an overall team third-order process. These second-order processes include actions conducted between performances (ie, transition processes), actions that occur as the team works toward a goal (ie, action processes), and actions focusing on the management of interpersonal relations (ie, interpersonal processes). Team effectiveness and member satisfaction are equally related to each of these three processes. In other words, all three second-order processes of team activities are each important in providing wanted outcomes and creating a sense of fulfillment among members.

How do HRTs effectively implement these second-order team processes? Decades of research into the characteristics of HRTs has spawned multiple models for team behavior and performance.[41] The Salas and colleagues[42] concept of The Big Five Model of Teamwork is particularly useful for identifying the key competencies needed to promote highly reliable team function. In it, they have identified five core individual-based behaviors common to HRTs that are successfully implemented using three key coordinating behaviors (**Table 2**).[5,39,41–43] These behaviors in turn can be categorized into team-based knowledge, skills, and attitudes (KSAs).[39] Additionally, Wilson and colleagues[43] mapped how these eight essential components relate to critical components of HROs, facilitating the development of effective training methods for creating HRTs and promoting a culture of safety within the team structure and organization.

What team-based competencies are applicable to the OR team? Clearly, the Big five core components and their coordinating mechanisms would play a role in any attempt to create HRTs within the OR. Nonetheless, each profession's particular roles and responsibilities in the OR might favor particular behaviors (ie, NTS) over others for effective team interaction. Fortunately, work from the Industrial Psychology Research Center at the University of Aberdeen has identified those key behavioral markers of NTS that are required by each profession in the OR for HRT performance (**Table 3**).[2,41,44–46] Although slightly different from the Big five behaviors, they can be roughly aligned. By identifying those NTS related to each profession in the OR, the development of targeted rating systems is possible for assessment of each profession.[46,47] Finally, by using the conceptual framework of the Big Five Model of Teamwork, accurate performance measures can be developed for assessing the effectiveness of training interventions.[41]

Approaching the OR team from the human factors perspective, therefore, reveals that it has the potential to be either a huge liability or an invaluable asset to the clinical microsystem and larger health care organization within which it functions. According to the University of Texas Medical Threat and Error Management Model proposed by Helmreich and Sexton,[48] the OR, like any clinical microsystem, should be viewed as an environment filled with both external threats (ie, unexpected events like an equipment failure) as well as latent threats (ie, overemphasis on case throughput) that, if not successfully identified and mitigated by the OR team, can lead to adverse events. Within this threat-filled environment work humans whose individual-based weaknesses (ie, limited memory, finite mental processing capacity, and susceptibility to stress or fatigue) predispose them to error production. In addition, group-based deficits such as *flawed teamwork* or negative cultural influences contribute to the generation of errors. To counteract such threats and errors, Helmreich and Sexton[48] have emphasized the development of a carefully designed program for change process, including training to improve teamwork. The challenge then becomes developing effective strategies for a surgical team training program.

STRATEGIES FOR SURGICAL TEAM TRAINING

Like any educational endeavor, developing an effective surgical team training program begins with the creation of a robust objectives-driven curriculum derived from targeted team-based KSAs (ie, competencies) identified through a thorough needs analysis of the learner group.[49,50] Clearly, content geared toward creating and promoting HRTs is desirable.[43] It should also use a human factors approach to error generation and team function as well as include training in behavioral countermeasures to threat and error (eg, inquiry, conflict resolution, and fatigue management).[48] Finally, the curricular content should attempt to introduce established tools for improving team

Table 2
The Big five model of teamwork—characteristics of core components and coordinating mechanisms in highly reliable teams

Category	Team-based Competency	Definition	Competency Type	Example	HRO Trait Equivalent(s)
Big 5 core components	Team leadership	Promotion of coordinated team performance through social problem solving and facilitation of goal definition and attainment	Skill	Assignment of roles to team members	Deference to expertise; reluctance to simplify
	Mutual performance monitoring	Keeping track of other members' work while performing own work	Skill	Providing feedback to promote self-correction	Commitment to resilience
	Back-up behavior	Shifting of workload among members in discretionary fashion to achieve balance	Skill	Completion of task by other team members with task saturation of an individual	Commitment to resilience
	Adaptability	Recognizing and appropriately responding to unexpected events or needs	Skill	Maintaining vigilance regarding cues of change in the course of events	Reluctance to simplify; preoccupation with failure
	Team orientation	Belief in the importance of the team's goals over individual goals	Attitude	Taking into account other team members' input	Deference to expertise; preoccupation with failure
Coordinating mechanisms	Shared mental model	A shared understanding of the situation and team goals for accomplishing objective	Knowledge	Implicit task coordination during high-workload situation	Commitment to resilience; reluctance to simplify; sensitivity to operations
	Mutual trust	Belief that team members will perform goals and protect each others' interests	Attitude	Admitting mistakes and accepting feedback regarding improvement	Deference to expertise; preoccupation with failure
	Communication	Exchange of information between sender and receiver	Skill	Initiation of message by sender, acknowledgment by receiver, follow-up by sender	Sensitivity to operations

Data from Refs. 5,39,41–43

Table 3
Profession-based behavioral markers of nontechnical skills (NTS) in the operating room

Skill Type	Nontechnical Skill	Profession	Proposed Big 5 Counterpart(s)
Cognitive	Situation awareness	Surgery	Shared mental model
		Anesthesia	Mutual performance monitoring
		Nursing	Adaptability
	Decision making	Surgery	Adaptability
		Anesthesia	
	Task management	Surgery	Adaptability
		Anesthesia	Mutual performance monitoring
Interpersonal	Leadership	Surgery	Team Leadership
	Communication	Surgery	Communication
		Nursing	
	Teamwork	Surgery	Team orientation
		Anesthesia	Mutual trust
		Nursing	Back-up behavior

Data from Refs.[2,41,44–46]

function (eg, standardized briefings, debriefing techniques, establishment of critical language, and assertiveness measures).[51]

Once created, a team training curriculum can then be implemented using a variety of instructional formats. Although a lecture-style format for mass distribution can be successfully implemented,[52] using a simulation-based training (SBT) format involving smaller groups of learners is best suited for ensuring transfer of team-based competencies to the actual clinical setting.[50] Ideally, SBT should target and involve the entire team unit to foster both cultural change within the organization and HRT function within the team itself.[43,53]

SBT can run the gamut of methodologies, each with varying levels of fidelity, cost, and optimal learner capacity (**Fig. 1**).[54–56] In addition, it can use a variety of instructional strategies to maximize training effectiveness and HRT function (**Table 4**).[43,50,57] Of the various SBT methodologies, team-centered HFS is particularly attractive because it creates a realistic and safe learning environment for practicing skills, managing rare events (eg, malignant hyperthermia), and revealing the consequences of team actions (eg, the natural course of an adverse event).[55] In HFS, fidelity is best achieved through mimicking the look and feel of the work system (ie, establishing equipment fidelity), re-creating the sensory cues of that system (ie, maintaining environment fidelity), and, most importantly, convincing the participants to "suspend disbelief" (ie, creating psychological fidelity).[55]

Like other forms of SBT, HFS is well suited for using a scenario-based training strategy for teaching team-based competencies. Rosen and colleagues[58] proposed using the event-based approach to training (EBAT) for such scenario development to create a standardized, structured learning experience for evaluating overall team and individual member performance. Key components of EBAT include defining specific learning objectives related to targeted teamwork competencies, framing the scenario development within a chosen clinical context, identifying KSAs related to the learning objectives, defining critical events and targeted responses related to the KSAs, creating appropriate measurement tools based on the targeted responses, and developing a scenario script.

Although robust scenario development using a structured methodology like EBAT is important, the debriefing is the critical teaching component of any HFS session. As a facilitative discussion among participants, it should focus on the strengths and

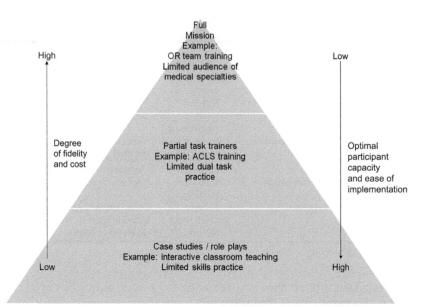

High

Low

Full
Mission
Example:
OR team training
Limited audience of
medical specialties

Degree
of fidelity
and cost

Optimal
participant
capacity
and ease of
implementation

Partial task trainers
Example: ACLS training
Limited dual task
practice

Case studies / role plays
Example: interactive classroom teaching
Limited skills practice

Low

High

Fig. 1. Simulation-based techniques used for team training. The pyramid demonstrates the interplay between level of fidelity, cost, optimal learner capacity, and ease of implementation among the various methodologies available for simulation-based training. With higher fidelity, costs increase whereas optimal participant capacity and ease of implementation decrease. ACLS, advanced cardiac life support. (*Data from* Paige JT, Chauvin S. Transforming the operating room through simulation training. Semin Colon Rectal Surg 2008;19:98–107; Beaubien JM, Baker DP. The use of simulation for training teamwork skills in health care: how low can you go? Qual Saf Health Care 2004;13:51–6; Frankel AS, Leonard MW, Denham CR. Fair and just culture, team behavior, and leadership engagement: the tools to achieve high reliability. Health Serv Res 2006;41:1691–709).

weaknesses of both the team and system that are revealed during the HFS scenario training.[59] An emphasis on "what is right" over "who is right" is critical in this setting of immediate feedback because it helps participants become more aware of patient care hazards and gives them the opportunity to help find solutions.[50,58] A debriefing facilitator capable of creating a safe environment in which learning objectives are met and in which participants focus on such processes as team communication and coordination is critical.[50]

Even though HFS-based team training is expensive and labor intensive, it can benefit learners at every point along the professional education continuum (ie, as student, resident, and practitioner).[56] Interprofessional HFS OR team training began in the 1990s in Basel, Switzerland, when clinicians from the OR departments at the Kantonsspital teamed up with investigators from the Human Factors Research Project at the University of Texas at Austin to create Team-Oriented Medical Simulation (TOMS).[60,61] Although this program is no longer functioning, interprofessional HFS OR team training has grown in popularity and has now been successfully implemented within specialized simulation centers[62–64] and at the point of care.[65–67] Distributed training of interprofessional OR teams using HFS has a demonstrated utility in reinforcing and expanding participants' positive attitudinal changes toward team-based competencies.[68]

Implementing an HFS-based training program can at first seem a rather daunting challenge. Developing a systematic approach to marshalling support, resources,

Table 4
Instructional strategies for simulation-based team training

Instructional Strategies	Proven Effectiveness in Team Training
Assertiveness training to model assertive/ nonassertive techniques	√
Meta-cognitive training to stimulate thinking about decision-making processes	√
Team coordination training	√
Cross-training	√
Perceptual contrast training to contrast positive and negative behaviors	√
Self-correction training to learn feedback processes	√
Guided error training to encourage problem solving through embedded errors	√
Scenario-based training using scripted scenarios to trigger behaviors	√

Data from Refs.[43,50,57]

and personnel is crucial for success. Paige[69] has proposed the "5P" approach, which attempts to group potential challenges into 5 major categories: finding a *patron*, developing a *plan*, locating a *place*, assembling the appropriate *people*, and choosing effective *products*. Both strategic and tactical solutions are then formulated to each one of these challenges. For example, developing a plan would entail the strategic creation of a robust curriculum as well as the tactical determination of such logistics as the scheduling of participants and the timing of sessions.

Does team training work? Salas and colleagues[57] remarked that, in general, all the previously mentioned team training strategies have been demonstrated to be effective in improving team cognitive, affective, process, and performance outcomes (see **Table 4**).[43,50,57] Cross training appears less effective than team coordination and guided self-correction training. Finally, every training strategy has been shown to have a positive influence on team functioning.

How effective is surgical team training? The introduction and adoption of something as simple as a preoperative protocol briefing has been demonstrated to positively affect team-based behaviors,[70,71] patient care process measures,[72] retention of personnel,[51] and surgical outcomes.[73] More structured didactic programs have demonstrated improved teamwork climate,[7] better communication among team members,[74] and more positive perceptions regarding teamwork.[75] HFS-based OR team training has been demonstrated to improve team-based attitudes among participants[67] as well as team-based behaviors within the actual OR.[76] It has also been successfully used to evaluate differences in team-based NTS among OR personnel[62] as well as "seasoned" and younger surgeons.[77] Such findings indicate that surgical team training is an effective modality for improving teamwork as well as the quality of patient care.

SUMMARY

Within today's complex, dynamic systems of health care, surgeons must draw on more than their technical skills to succeed. Instead, they must bring key NTS to bear to promote team-based competencies within the OR team and to ensure its cohesive function. By endorsing a human factors perspective to organizational culture, error generation, and team-based science, surgeons can identify and adopt effective surgical team training strategies for incorporation into an objectives-driven training program based on key team-based competencies. In this manner, they will assist in the transformation of the dysfunctional OR teams of the present into the highly reliable OR teams of the future.

REFERENCES

1. Ericsson KA. Deliberate practice and the acquisition and maintenance of expert performance in medicine and related domains. Acad Med 2004;79(10):S70–81.
2. Fletcher GCL, McGeorge P, Flin RH, et al. The role of non-technical skills in anesthesia: a review of current literature. Br J Anaesth 2002;88:418–29.
3. North Carolina State University Counseling Center. Interpersonal skills. Available at: http://www.ncsu.edu/counseling_center/resources/personal/interpersonal_skills/interpersonal_skills.htm. Accessed October 31, 2009.
4. Flin R, Martin L, Goeters K, et al. Development of the NOTECHS (Non-technical skills) system for assessing pilots' CRM skills. Human Factors and Aerospace Safety 2003;3:95–117.
5. Baker DP, Day R, Salas E. Teamwork as an essential component of high-reliability organizations. Health Serv Res 2006;41:1576–98.
6. Burke CS, Salas E, Wilson-Donnelly K, et al. How to turn a team of experts into an expert medical team: guidance from the aviation and military communities. Qual Saf Health Care 2004;13(Suppl 1):i96–i104.
7. Bleakley A, Boyden J, Hobbs A, et al. Improving teamwork climate in operating theatres: the shift from multiprofessionalism to interprofessionalism. J Interprof Care 2006;20(5):461–70.
8. Bleakley A. You are who I say you are: the rhetorical construction of identity in the operating theatre. J Workplace Learning 2006;18(7–8):414–25.
9. Helmreich RL, Merritt AC. In: Culture at work in aviation and medicine: national, organizational, and professional influences. Aldershot (UK): Ashgate; 1998. p. 27–52.
10. McDonald R, Waring J, Harrison S, et al. Rules and guidelines in clinical practice: a qualitative study in operating theatres of doctors' and nurses' views. Qual Saf Health Care 2005;14:290–4.
11. Undre S, Sevdalis N, Healy AN, et al. Teamwork in the operating theatre: cohesion or confusion? J Eval Clin Pract 2006;12:182–9.
12. Lingard L, Reznick R, DeVito I, et al. Forming professional identities on the health care team: discursive constructions of the 'other' in the operating room. Med Educ 2002;36:728–34.
13. Flin R, Yule S, McKenzie L, et al. Attitudes to teamwork and safety in the operating theatre. Surgeon 2006;4:145–51.
14. Moorthy K, Munz Y, Adams S, et al. Imperial College –St. Mary's Hospital Simulation Group. Self-assessment of performance among surgical trainees during simulated procedures in a simulated operating theater. Am J Surg 2006;192:114–8.
15. Paige JT, Aaron DL, Yang T, et al. Implementation of a preoperative briefing protocol improves accuracy of teamwork assessment in the operating room. Am Surg 2008;79:817–23.
16. Makary MA, Sexton JB, Freischlag JA, et al. Operating room teamwork among physicians and nurses: teamwork in the eye of the beholder. J Am Coll Surg 2006;202:746–52.

17. Lingard L, Espin S, Whyte S, et al. Communication failures in the operating room: an observational classification of recurrent types and effects. Qual Saf Health Care 2004;13:330–4.
18. Lingard L, Garwood S, Poenaru D. Tensions influencing operating room team function: does institutional context make a difference? Med Educ 2004;38:691–9.
19. Helmrich RL, Davies JM. Team performance in the operating room. In: Bogner MS, editor. Human error in medicine. Hillside (NJ): Erlbaum; 1994. p. 225–53.
20. Nestel D, Kidd JM. Nurses' perceptions and experiences of communication in the operating theatre: a focus group interview. BMC Nurs 2006;5:1.
21. Rosenstein AH, O'Daniel M. Impact and implications of disruptive behavior in the perioperative arena. J Am Coll Surg 2006;203:96–105.
22. Christian CK, Gustafson ML, Roth EM, et al. A prospective study of patient safety in the operating room. Surgery 2006;139:159–73.
23. Mishra A, Catchpole K, Dale T, et al. The influence of non-technical performance on technical outcome in laparoscopic cholecystectomy. Surg Endosc 2008;22:68–73.
24. Joint Commission on Accreditation of Healthcare Organizations. Root causes of wrong site surgery. Available at: http://www.jointcommission.org/NR/rdonlyres/90B92D9B-9D55-4469-94B1-DA64A8147F74/0/se_rc_wss.jpg. Accessed October 31, 2009.
25. Kwaan MR, Studdert DM, Zinner MJ, et al. Incidence, patterns, and prevention or wrong-site surgery. Arch Surg 2006;141:352–7.
26. Greenberg CC, Regenbogen SE, Studdert DM, et al. Patterns of communication breakdowns resulting in injury to surgical patients. J Am Coll Surg 2007;204: 533–40.
27. Mazzocco K, Petitti DB, Fong KT, et al. Surgical team behaviors and patient outcomes. Am J Surg 2009;197:678–85.
28. Gawron VJ, Drury CG, Fairbanks RJ, et al. Medical error and human factors engineering: where are we now? Am J Med Qual 2006;21:57–67.
29. Reason J. Human error: models and management. BMJ 2000;320:768–70.
30. Reason J. Safety in the operating theatre—part 2: human error and organizational failure. Qual Saf Health Care 2005;14:56–61.
31. Reason J. In: Managing the risks of organizational accidents. Aldershot (UK): Ashgate; 1997. p. 1–20.
32. Mohr JJ, Batalden PB. Improving safety on the frontline: the role of the clinical microsystem. Qual Saf Health Care 2002;11:45–50.
33. Westrum R. A typology of organizational cultures. Qual Saf Health Care 2004;12: 22–7.
34. Carroll JS, Quijada MA. Redirecting traditional professional values to support safety: changing organizational culture in health care. Qual Saf Health Care 2004;13(Suppl II):ii16–21.
35. Singer SJ, Gaba DM, Geppert JJ, et al. The culture of safety: results of an organization-wide survey in 15 California hospitals. Qual Saf Health Care 2003;12: 112–8.
36. Schulman PR. General attributes of safe organizations. Qual Saf Health Care 2004;13(Suppl II):ii39–44.
37. McKeon LM, Oswaks JD, Cunningham PD. Safeguarding patients: complexity science, high reliability organizations, and implications for team training in healthcare. Clin Nurse Spec 2006;20:298–304.
38. Katzenbach JR, Smith DK. In: The wisdom of teams. New York: HarperCollins; 2003. p. 87–109.

39. Baker DP, Gustafson S, Beaubien J, et al. Medical teamwork and patient safety: the evidence-based relation. AHRQ Publication No. 05–0053. Rockville (MD): Agency for Healthcare Research and Quality; April 2005. Available at: http://www.ahrq.gov/qual/medteam/. Accessed October 31, 2009.

40. LePine JA, Piccolo RF, Jackson CL, et al. A meta-analysis of teamwork processes: tests of a multi-dimensional model and relationships with team effectiveness criteria. Personnel Psych 2008;61:273–307.

41. Salas E, Rosen MA, Held JD, et al. Performance measurement in simulation-based training: a review and best practices. Simul Gaming 2009;40:328–76.

42. Salas E, Sims DE, Burke CS. Is there a big five in teamwork? Small Gr Res 2005; 36:555–99.

43. Wilson KA, Burke CS, Priest HA, et al. Promoting health care safety through training high reliability teams. Qual Saf Health Care 2005;14:303–9.

44. Yule S, Flin R, Paterson-Brown S, et al. Non-technical skills for surgeons in the operating room: a review of the literature. Surgery 2006;139:140–9.

45. Mitchell L, Flin R. Non-technical skills of the operating theatre scrub nurse: a literature review. J Adv Nurs 2008;63:15–24.

46. Yule S, Flin R, Paterson-Brown S, et al. Development of a rating system for surgeons' non-technical skills. Med Educ 2006;40:1098–104.

47. Fletcher G, Flin R, McGeorge P, et al. Rating non-technical skills: developing a behavioural marker system for use in anaesthesia. Cognit Tech Work 2004;6: 165–71.

48. Helmreich RL, Sexton JB. Managing threat and error to increase safety in medicine. In: Dietrich R, Jochum K, editors. Teaming up: components of safety under high risk. Aldershot (UK): Ashgate; 2004. p. 115–32.

49. Rosen MA, Salas E, Wilson KA, et al. Measuring team performance in simulation-based training: adopting best practices for healthcare. Sim Healthcare 2008;3:33–41.

50. Fernandez R, Vozenilek JA, Hegarty CB, et al. Developing expert medical teams: toward an evidence-based approach. Acad Emerg Med 2008;15:1025–36.

51. Leonard M, Graham S, Bonacum D. The human factor: the critical importance of effective teamwork and communication in providing safe care. Qual Saf Health Care 2004;13(Suppl I):i85–90.

52. Grogan EL, Stiles RA, France DJ, et al. The impact of aviation-based teamwork training on the attitudes of health-care professionals. J Am Coll Surg 2004;199:843–8.

53. Firth-Cozens J. Cultures for improving patient safety through learning: the role of teamwork. Qual Saf Health Care 2001;10(Suppl II):ii26–31.

54. Paige JT, Chauvin S. Transforming the operating room through simulation training. Semin Colon Rectal Surg 2008;19:98–107.

55. Beaubien JM, Baker DP. The use of simulation for training teamwork skills in health care: how low can you go? Qual Saf Health Care 2004;13:51–6.

56. Frankel AS, Leonard MW, Denham CR. Fair and just culture, team behavior, and leadership engagement: the tools to achieve high reliability. Health Serv Res 2006;41:1691–709.

57. Salas E, DiazGrandos D, Weaver SJ, et al. Does team training work? Principles of health care. Acad Emerg Med 2008;15:1002–9.

58. Rosen MA, Salas E, Wu TS, et al. Promoting teamwork: an event-based approach to simulation-based teamwork training for emergency medicine residents. Acad Emerg Med 2008;15:1190–8.

59. Hamman W. In-situ simulation: using aviation principles to identify relevant teamwork and systems issues to promote patient safety. Harvard International Journal 2008;26:9–11.

60. Sexton B, Marsch S, Helmreich R, et al. Participant evaluation of team oriented medical simulation. Available at: http://homepage.psy.utexas.edu/homepage/group/HelmreichLAB/Publications/226.doc. Accessed October 31, 2009.
61. Betzenderfer D. Anesthesia Patient Safety Foundation. Available at: http://www.apsf.org/resource_center/newsletter/1996/spring/apsfled_betzen.html. Accessed October 31, 2009.
62. Undre S, Koutantji M, Sevdalis N, et al. Multidisciplinary crisis simulations: the way forward for training surgical teams. World J Surg 2007;31:1843–53.
63. Paige JT, Kozmenko V, Morgan B, et al. From the flight deck to the operating room: impact of a simulation based interdisciplinary team training pilot program in crisis management. J Surg Ed 2007;64(6):369–77.
64. Powers KA, Rehrig ST, Irias N, et al. Simulated laparoscopic operating room crisis: an approach to enhance the surgical team performance. Surg Endosc 2008;22:885–900.
65. Paige JT, Kozmenko V, Yang T, et al. The mobile mock operating room: bringing team training to the point of care. Advances in patient safety: new directions and alternative approaches. In: Performance and tools, vol. 3. AHRQ Publication Nos. 08-0034. (1-4). Rockville (MD): Agency for Healthcare Research and Quality; 2008. Available at: http://www.ahrq.gov/qual/advances2/. Accessed October 31, 2009.
66. Flanagan B, Joseph M, Bujor M, et al. Attitudes to safety and teamwork in the operating theatre, and the effects of a program of simulation-based team training. In: Anca JM Jr, editor. Multimodal safety management and human factors. Aldershot (UK): Ashgate; 2007. p. 211–20.
67. Paige JT, Kozmenko V, Yang T, et al. High-fidelity, simulation-based, interdisciplinary operating room team training at the point of care. Surgery 2009;145(2):138–46.
68. Paige JT, Kozmenko V, Yang T, et al. Attitudinal changes resulting from repetitive training of operating room personnel using high-fidelity simulation at the point-of-care. Am Surg 2009;75(7):584–91.
69. Paige JT, Team training at the point of care. In: Tsuda S, Scott DJ, Jones DB, editors. Textbook of simulation, surgical skills, and team training. Woodbury: Cine-Med, Inc; in press.
70. Lingard L, Regehr G, Orser B, et al. Evaluation of a preoperative checklist and team briefing among surgeons, nurses, and anesthesiologists to reduce failures in communication. Arch Surg 2008;143:12–7.
71. Paige JT, Aaron DL, Yang T, et al. Improved operating room teamwork via SAFETY Prep: a rural community hospital's experience. World J Surg 2009;33(6):1181–7.
72. Altpeter T, Luckhardt K, Lewis JN, et al. Expanded surgical time out: a key to real-time data collection and quality improvement. J Am Coll Surg 2007;204:527–32.
73. Haynes AB, Weiser TG, Berry WR, , et alSafe Surgery Saves Lives Study Group. A surgical safety checklist to reduce morbidity and mortality in a global population. N Engl J Med 2009;360(5):491–9.
74. Awad SS, Fagan SP, Bellows C, et al. Bridging the communication gap in the operating room with medical team training. Am J Surg 2005;190:770–4.
75. Halverson AL, Andersson JL, Anderson K, et al. Surgical team training: the Northwestern Memorial Hospital experience. Arch Surg 2009;144(2):107–12.
76. Paige JT, Kozmenko V, Yang T, et al. High fidelity, simulation-based training at the point-of-care improves teamwork in the operating room. J Am Coll Surg 2008; 207:S87–8.
77. Powers K, Rehrig ST, Schwaitzberg SD, et al. Seasoned surgeons assessed in a laparoscopic crisis. J Gastrointest Surg 2009;13(5):994–1003.

Optimizing Learning in Surgical Simulations: Guidelines from the Science of Learning and Human Performance

Janis A. Cannon-Bowers, PhD[a],*, Clint Bowers, PhD[b],
Katelyn Procci, BS[b]

KEYWORDS

• Simulation • Optimization • Feedback • Cognition • Training

At this point in its evolution, the use of simulation to train surgeons has come of age. There are now numerous empirical investigations (in surgery and other areas) supporting the use of simulation technologies to teach various surgical competencies. Hence, we (the authors of this article) believe that it is no longer necessary to demonstrate that simulation can be a useful training tool for surgeons; the appropriate question to pose at this point is: how do we optimize learning through simulation? Consistent with other complex behavioral phenomena, this question does not have a simple, straightforward answer. Instead, research into training system design has consistently concluded that the effectiveness of any training technique depends on a host of factors, including characteristics of the learner, the learning objectives being trained, various features of the training system and learning environment, and the context in which training occurs.

All that said, we believe that it is possible to develop prescriptions about how best to design and implement simulation-based training in surgery by gleaning guidelines and lessons learned from the general science of learning literature, then using these to construct specific hypotheses about what will be successful for various surgical competencies. Such an approach allows practitioners to benefit immediately from the most current wisdom about simulation-based training, while setting the stage for a research agenda that represents a principled approach to evolving simulation-based surgical education (ie, that builds incrementally on what is already known

[a] Institute for Simulation & Training, University of Central Florida, 3100 Technology Parkway, Orlando, FL 32826, USA
[b] Department of Psychology, University of Central Florida, 4000 Central Florida Boulevard, Orlando, FL 32816, USA
* Corresponding author.
E-mail address: jancb@mail.ucf.edu

Surg Clin N Am 90 (2010) 583–603
doi:10.1016/j.suc.2010.02.006
0039-6109/10/$ – see front matter © 2010 Elsevier Inc. All rights reserved.

surgical.theclinics.com

and investigates potentially high-payoff interventions). Our goal in this article is to commence this process. Although we are unable to review and summarize the entire science of learning literature, we have selected aspects of it that we believe can have significant added value for surgical education.

To accomplish this goal, the organization of this article is as follows. First, we present a set of findings offered in 2005 by Issenberg and colleagues[1] that resulted from a comprehensive review of literature investigating the effectiveness of medical simulations. We chose these findings as a foundation on which to build because they resulted from a well-designed and rigorous review of the empirical literature into medical simulation. Next, we sample literature from the science of learning and human performance that can optimize the way in which selected features from the list by Issenberg and colleagues[1] are instantiated in surgical simulation. In doing so, we consider a host of features and variables that we believe have a high probability of positive impact. At the conclusion of each section, we summarize what we have reviewed into a set of actionable guidelines for practitioners. We close by delineating a set of research issues that we believe must be investigated as we move forward in simulation-based surgical simulation.

FEATURES OF EFFECTIVE TRAINING SIMULATIONS

Issenberg and colleagues[1] conducted a well-designed and rigorous review of the literature on medical simulations, with the goal of isolating the features that contribute most to their learning effectiveness. Completed as part of the Best Evidence Medical Education collaboration, this report systematically reviewed and coded 109 empirical articles and concluded that the following features appear to be most closely associated with simulator effectiveness:

- *Feedback* is provided during learning experience
- Learners engage in *repetitive practice*
- Simulator is integrated into the overall curriculum
- Learners practice with increasing *levels of difficulty*
- Adaptable to multiple *learning strategies*
- Clinical variation
- Controlled environment
- Individualized learning
- *Outcomes/benchmarks* clearly stated and tangible
- Validity of simulator.

Perhaps not surprisingly, many of these features are similar to those found in any effective instructional system. In fact, considerable research has been conducted into how to manipulate these features to optimize learning. Using these features as a starting point (particularly the ones shown in italics), we selected the following topics for review and summary in this article:

- Nature of feedback: when and how feedback should be delivered, optimal frequency of feedback
- Conditions of practice: best practice strategies and schedules
- Scenario design: systematically manipulating the difficulty and variability of scenarios
- Learning/instructional strategies: which learning strategies optimize learning within simulations, how to implement various learning strategies
- Goal setting: nature of goals that lead to highest performance and learning

- Performance measurement: elements of effective performance measures in training.

In addition, we highlight several other findings from the general science of learning literature that we believe have implications for the design of simulation-based surgical training. These findings fall under the general category of:

- *Pretraining motivation and expectations* — how these can be increased to ensure maximum learning.

The sections that follow address each of these topics, and conclude with a set of guidelines that can be implemented immediately as well as recommendations for research directions needed to address remaining questions.

FEEDBACK

Perhaps the most often-cited feature of instruction that fosters learning is feedback, and with good reason. According to many learning theorists, feedback is a primary mechanism by which learning occurs. For example, Gagne-Briggs' Theory of Instructional Design delineates the pivotal role of feedback in learning. According to this theory, effective feedback serves many purposes such as the following: focuses and maintains the attention of the trainee; outlines clear goals; draws on learned knowledge; provides guidance; initiates practice; and provides informative, contextual, and objective information.[2,3] In this sense, feedback is not a judgment but a behavioral correction that is necessary for the acquisition of new skills.[3] Hewson and Little[4] outline several other recommendations for effective feedback, generally stating that the best feedback is respectful and nonjudgmental, and is focused on specific behaviors with suggestions for future development and enhancement.

Despite the obvious importance of feedback in training, there is surprisingly little guidance about the optimum content or timing of feedback. In the following sections, we discuss the available research regarding these aspects of feedback and attempt to extract guidelines about how best to provide feedback in the specific case of surgical simulation.

Types of Feedback

There are 2 main types of feedback: process feedback and outcome feedback. Outcome feedback simply provides information about overall performance outcomes, akin to a final score. Process feedback is typically more specific, providing detailed information about the behavior and why it was correct or incorrect. Process feedback sometimes offers specific guidance on how to improve in subsequent performance. Each of these feedback types has strengths and weaknesses. For example, process feedback allows learners to draw immediate associations between their actions and the consequences of those actions. However, in high-workload training environments, this type of feedback may overwhelm the learner and actually detract from eventual learning. Process feedback can also prevent learners from seeing the natural consequences of their choices because correction is made before those consequences are manifested. On the other hand, outcome feedback may allow learners to maintain a suboptimal, or even completely incorrect, pattern of performance until the end of the practice trial. This pattern may lead to frustration and resentment, particularly because not all learners are able to discern a better course of action and may experience negative training.

Generally speaking, the early research literature suggested that process feedback is superior to outcome feedback unless the task is very simple or the learner is very experienced.[5,6] In fact, some investigators have suggested that outcome feedback alone can even impede long-term learning because trainees make incorrect attributions as to why their performance is deficient.[7]

However, much of the early research on feedback type focused largely on fairly simple cognitive tasks and emphasized short-term knowledge acquisition. More recently, researchers have begun to investigate the effects of various feedback types on other types of competencies and on longer term sustainment of knowledge and skills. These results have been somewhat less clear. For example, Korsgaard and Diddams[8] studied the effect of feedback type on decision-making performance. In simple problems, there was no advantage for any feedback type but for complex problems they found that outcome feedback was associated with much better performance than was a combination of outcome and process feedback. This finding supports the notion that process feedback might be overwhelming in complex tasks. However, this difference faded at the second trial, with each feedback type being equivalent.

Little research has been done on feedback for complex tasks that involve cognitive and psychomotor demands (which would be of particular interest for training surgical competencies). One might suspect that learners in these tasks are even more likely to be overwhelmed by the cognitive demands of process feedback. However, these tasks might also be the most difficult for the use of outcome feedback. There clearly is a need for much more research on the effects of the type of feedback provided to the learner in complex situations. In the meantime, there seems to be a small advantage for process feedback, especially for novice learners. However, this type of feedback should be provided with careful attention to the learner's cognitive load.

Timing and Frequency of Feedback

Turning first to the issue of optimal timing of feedback, there are 2 main views as to when feedback should be provided, either immediately after the behavior or after a delayed time interval. There are arguments for and against both temporal approaches. Immediate feedback has the apparent advantage of immediately correcting misconceptions. It has been suggested that this advantage increases the likelihood that the original, incorrect, belief can be changed in memory.[9] Further, Gibson[10] argues that it is necessary in dynamic environments to have immediate feedback as opposed to delayed feedback because delayed feedback means that corrections are not given within context. Alternatively, delayed feedback allows the learner to dedicate his or her entire attention (in most cases) to the feedback. It also reduces the likelihood that during-performance feedback becomes a "crutch" that reduces transfer.[11]

Overall, the research literature suggests that immediate feedback is associated with faster and better learning.[5,12] However, delayed feedback has typically been associated with greater long-term knowledge retention.[13,14] Specific studies of surgical skill training tend to mimic this pattern. For example, Xeroulis and colleagues[15] have reported on the effects of feedback timing on surgical knot-tying skill. These investigators report that immediate and delayed feedback lead to knowledge acquisition gains, but only delayed feedback is associated with sustained skill over time. Similar results were obtained with endoscopic surgery trainees.[16]

A related issue pertains to the frequency of feedback. Trainers have often believed that feedback must be provided after every performance episode in order for optimal learning to occur. However, it seems that the frequency of feedback influences learning and retention in a manner similar to the timing of feedback. That is, more frequent feedback seems to be associated with faster acquisition, whereas fewer feedback episodes are typically associated with greater retention.[17,18,19]

Other Issues Related to Feedback Delivery

Several other issues related to optimizing feedback are worth mentioning, the first of which is the modality used to present feedback. Specifically, in a visually complex and demanding task it may be possible to provide auditory feedback (eg, a tone or alarm when an error is made). The rationale here is that as the visual channel is likely overloaded, auditory feedback puts no extra burden on this already overloaded system. This view is consistent with multiple resource theory,[19] which posits that humans process information through a set of relatively independent channels. Hence, engaging multiple channels enhances the overall capacity of information that can be processed.

Regarding the delivery of the feedback itself, this should always be nonjudgmental and as objective as possible.[2] If trainees become defensive, they clearly are less likely to acquire targeted skills. This is an important concern, and simply assuming that instructors possess effective feedback delivery skills is unwise. In fact, it may be prudent to invest in instructor training that improves the quality of feedback delivery.

Guidelines

Based on the literature reviewed in this article, the following guidelines for delivering feedback are offered:

1. For novice learners, process feedback should be provided during the skill acquisition process.
2. Trainers should monitor the cognitive load of trainees and delay feedback during periods of heavy load.
3. Process feedback should gradually be faded in favor of outcome feedback.
4. Provide feedback after errors.
5. Consider delivering feedback in a separate channel from the one most overloaded by the task.
6. Delayed feedback should be used in surgical simulation, particularly for more advanced learners.
7. Technology should be used to recreate the context of the feedback to assist in the assimilation of the feedback.
8. Instructors should be trained in how to deliver effective feedback.

CONDITIONS OF PRACTICE

Football coach Vince Lombardi amended the old adage "practice makes perfect" to "perfect practice makes perfect." From a learning and human performance standpoint, the amended version seems to fit empirical findings related to the relationship between practice and learning. Specifically, various approaches to structuring practice sessions have been investigated, and some clearly have advantages over others. The sections that follow briefly review these findings.

Part- Versus Whole-Task Practice

The popular instructional design model proposed by van Merriënboer and colleagues[20] posits that novices learn complex tasks differently than they learn simple tasks. According to this model, learning complex tasks requires the development of schema (or mental models), which are general strategies or scripts that direct behavior. van Merriënboer and colleagues argue that when a complex task is broken down into small parts and learning is sequenced, the result is a set of nonintegrated steps or procedures. Conversely, when the entire task is learned at once, all steps of the task can be coordinated and integrated within the appropriate context. Hence, dynamic problem solving is more efficient because there are established schema for reference as opposed to a set of nonintegrated steps.

An example of a study pitting whole- versus part-task training was conducted by Lim and Reiser.[21] Specifically, this study investigated the impact of whole- or part-task instruction on the learning of complex cognitive skills and transfer of training. The investigators found that those in the whole-task condition performed better than those in the part-task condition on a posttraining achievement test. One explanation for this finding might be that those in the whole-task condition had more opportunities to integrate the skills they learned, and were therefore able to perform parts of the task and the whole task more efficiently. Lim and Reiser also argued that enhanced schema creation may have led to long-lasting retention in a contextually correct environment.

Although there is considerable support for the notion that whole-task practice benefits learning for complex tasks,[22,23] some research continues to support the traditional part-task learning methodology. For example, one study concerning a computer simulation training program that taught aircrews to estimate the location and spatial orientation of aircraft found that those in the part-task condition engaged in more practice sessions than those in the whole-task condition; those who were taught using whole-task methodology performed more poorly than those in the part-task condition and took more time to complete the training program.[23]

One problem with whole-task instruction is the management of cognitive load. Particularly when dealing with complex tasks, the nature of whole-task instruction often leads to high cognitive load. With simple learning tasks, the amount of cognitive load may not be an issue.[24] High cognitive load during complex task training, in turn, can be detrimental to overall learning and performance.[25] This finding is explained by the cognitive resource theory, which posits that only a limited amount of information can be processed at one time. By limiting cognitive load, there are more resources available to engage in the learning process, resulting in improved training outcomes.[24]

Although complex tasks inherently impose higher cognitive load than simpler tasks, it is also the case that as an individual gains competence, cognitive load decreases because aspects of performance become automatic. Following this line of reasoning, it would seem prudent to use a whole-task approach with novices only when the task can be simplified enough to not overwhelm trainees. Later in training, it makes sense to present the entire problem when learners are better able to cope with the complexity.

Practice Schedules

Establishing a practice schedule is another aspect of instructional design that is vital to the success of any training system. There are 2 main types of practice schedules, defined temporally as spaced and massed training. Spaced training involves distributing learning tasks and skill acquisition practice sessions over a specified time interval, whereas massed practice occurs over the course of 1 or 2 intense and content-heavy sessions.[26]

A well-developed body of literature suggests that spaced practice is superior over massed practice for long-term retention.[26,27,28] A meta-analysis conducted by Cepeda and colleagues[29] found that performance using spaced as opposed to massed practice was improved by 9%. However, this effect seems to hold for long-term retention (or transfer); for short-term retention, massed practice seems to be better than spaced.[30] According to Schmidt and Bjork,[11] the explanation for this seems to be similar to the explanation for providing less feedback in training. Specifically, these researchers (and others) argue that creating difficulties for the learner in the acquisition phase seems to lead to increased long-term retention and transfer (at the expense of short-term performance).

The issue of exactly how long-spaced practice intervals need to be is probably dependent on the nature of the task and level of learners. In a study related to learning a foreign language, Bahrick and colleagues[31] found that longer time intervals between practice sessions resulted in increased retention despite slower acquisition rates. For the first year, retention was best for those in the 14-day time interval; however, after that time frame those individuals in the 56-day interval condition had the best retention rates for the subsequent years up until the fifth year. Pashler and colleagues[28] go as far as suggesting that to maintain information in the long term, the time intervals between practice sessions should consist of longer periods (months to years) as opposed to shorter periods, and that too little spacing might even be detrimental to learning.

Guidelines for Structuring Practice

1. Employ part-task practice strategies early in learning for complex tasks
2. If the task can be simplified, whole-task practice can be appropriate for novices
3. Use whole-task practice strategies for more advanced learners
4. Employ a spaced-practice approach to maximize long-term retention
5. Consider refresher training, spaced over months and years, to ensure long-term retention.

SCENARIO DESIGN

Several of the features of effective simulation noted by Issenberg and colleagues[1] are related to the design of cases or scenarios presented within the simulation. In fact, the design of effective, appropriate scenarios is one of the most crucial issues involved in simulation-based training.[32] According to Cannon-Bowers and Bowers,[33] the scenario is the mechanism by which learning objectives are exercised and essentially constitute the curriculum when using simulation as the instructional method.

Medical educators typically use the term "case" instead of scenario (which is used by training researchers). The primary difference between what is typically meant by a case and what training researchers call a scenario seems to be that cases often do not contain an ongoing timeline (ie, the pertinent facts are presented once at the beginning of the case) and they are often not interactive in the sense that they change or branch in response to the learners' input (although they are interactive in the sense that they are often used as the basis for a discussion or didactic exchange). This is not to say that cases are not used in more interactive ways, just that they often are not the basis of an interactive, performance-based experience. The rapid maturity of technologies that allows presentation of computerized or digital cases (ie, using avatars instead of mannequins or standardized patients) may change this.

With respect to developing effective scenarios, several researchers have conceptualized this process in terms of embedding specific events into scenarios that represent the learning objectives. According to Cannon-Bowers,[34] an event (in this context) is "any stimulus condition that is purposely scripted into a scenario to elicit a particular response." Scenario events have also been conceptualized as triggers, specific scenario conditions that allow the trainee to practice the targeted learning objectives[35,36] as a means to demonstrate proficiency and/or as a basis for feedback. Hence, the scenario events form the basis of trainee practice opportunities. To date, the event-based approach to training has been successfully demonstrated in several settings.[36,37]

Scenario design in simulation-based systems must also consider the level of challenge in trigger events or activities. Incorporating challenges into learning has motivational benefits; however, challenges that are beyond the capability of trainees may also be frustrating and actually impair progress. According to Kozlowski and colleagues,[38] evidence also suggests that variability in scenario or problem design is important to ensure adequate long-term transfer of skills. That is, paying attention to the ways in which the task varies in the real world and representing these in scenarios should benefit performance. Moreover, providing variations of a problem or case helps to build robust schema or mental models that can help them adapt to novel situations when they occur. This contention was borne out in the Issenberg and colleagues[1] study, which found that clinical variation was a characteristic of effective surgical simulations. In addition, Kozlowski and colleagues[38] recommend that in environments where errors are a frequent occurrence in the real task environment, difficult problems in training allow trainees to make errors and practice problem-solving skills necessary to develop error-coping strategies.

The scenario in simulation-based training can also serve another purpose; that is, to provide a context or narrative in which individual events or triggers can be tied together. For certain types of simulations—for example, those that involve team-level objectives or interacting with patients throughout the continuum of care—the "back story" needs to anchor and provide a context for the learning events. In this sense, the scenario or story can also serve a motivational purpose because it engages the trainee in a realistic context. Researchers are beginning to theorize that narrative elements may actually enhance learning by helping to guide trainees through the system.[20] Recent research also suggests that psychological concepts such as immersion and presence—which can be increased through compelling narrative—may enhance learning because trainees are psychologically engaged in the scenario.[21] The narrative or story can also contribute to the authenticity of the experiences trainees gain in training; that is, the extent to which they are rich, faithful representations of the world that will enable the trainee to transfer his/her virtual experience into the real environment. This whole includes the affective or emotional aspects as well as more cognitive and behavioral factors.

Guidelines for Scenario Design

1. Script scenarios deliberately to ensure that targeted material is covered.
2. Construct trigger events in scenarios that address each learning objective directly.
3. Script several trigger events that target the same learning objectives either in a single scenario or in multiple scenarios.
4. Develop trigger events that provide challenge to learners without overwhelming them.
5. Develop scenarios with increasing challenges scripted into trigger events.
6. Create a narrative (back story) that is engaging to trainees and that can incorporate trigger events.
7. Script variability into trigger events that represent different manifestations of the problem.

LEARNING/INSTRUCTIONAL STRATEGIES

It has long been recognized that simulators or simulation-based training provides a vehicle or context in which learning can occur. To optimize learning, training researchers have investigated a variety of strategies that can be implemented within a simulation-based environment. Although these strategies range widely in how and when they are implemented, they are all designed to make best use of simulation environment. We have selected several for discussion in this article.

Attentional Advice

Simulation-based training is often characterized by complex problems presented in stimulus-rich environments. As noted, this complexity runs the risk of imposing a high-level of extraneous cognitive load.[39] It is feared by some theorists in this area that this extraneous load may redirect cognitive resources from the main task of learning, especially in novice or low-ability learners.[40] Although there are specific factors related to the training itself that can be manipulated to avoid extraneous load,[41] it has been suggested that cognitive load can also be managed through the use of pretraining interventions designed to direct the trainees' attention. A common method of accomplishing this is a pretraining briefing through which the goals of training are articulated along with guidance about how to direct one's effort in the upcoming training exercise.

Other researchers have labeled this type of guidance attentional advice.[42] The research data indicate that this type of guidance can be useful for helping trainees identify crucial problem elements and direct their attention accordingly.[43] In summary, merely telling trainees the elements to which they should attend is likely to improve their learning, especially in complex scenarios.

Advance Organizers

Learning scientists maintain that learning new material imposes several cognitive demands on learners. Not only must they identify, extract, and understand new material, but must also infer the relationships between items and organize knowledge on the fly. It has been suggested that trainers can reduce some of these demands by providing advance organizers.[44] Advance organizers originally were presented as text passages designed to provide an organizational schema to assist with assimilating new knowledge. However, since that time researchers have used any number of graphical, text, animated, or mixed presentation schemes.

There is extensive literature on the effects of advance organizers. Like any large body of research, there are contradictory results. However, most reviews and meta-analyses have concluded that there are mild to moderate positive effects for these interventions.[45] Consequently, researchers have turned their attention to identifying the specific modes of presentation of advance organizers that optimize knowledge transfer. For example, there has been considerable research investigating text versus graphical advance organizer approaches. Generally speaking, the data favor the use of graphical presentations, especially when the material involves understanding relationships between relatively unlike constructs.[39] Combined text and graphic presentations can also be useful in many situations.[46,47] The particular format that is optimal for a particular training situation probably depends on the nature and complexity of the task being trained. What seems to be most important is that the advance organizer helps the learner to develop knowledge structures that are robust and well structured to allow for incorporation of subsequent learning content.

Examples/Worked-Out Examples

Another instructional strategy that has been studied is the use of examples in training, especially worked-out examples that describe the solution and how it was arrived at by an expert. In this regard, Anderson and Schunn[48] argue that a primary mechanism for learners to acquire procedural knowledge is by the use of examples. This view holds that when a learner is presented with a novel problem (and hence has a goal to solve the problem), he or she needs to be shown an example of the solution (or he/she will be forced to attempt a solution through trial and error). Anderson and Schunn contend further that to be successful, the example must be understood by the learner in terms of its relevance to the current problem and what exactly is being conveyed. These requirements mean that the explanations that accompany examples in learning must be clear, detailed, and understandable, while highlighting the crucial similarities and differences between the current problem and preceding ones.

The use of worked-out examples, in which learners are given an example of a problem that has been solved by an expert, has also been studied extensively. According to Sweller and colleagues,[49] learning effectiveness and efficiency are enhanced when worked-out examples are substituted for practice problems because they reduce the cognitive load on the user.[50] However, recent studies indicate that this effect holds for trainees with less prior knowledge in a domain (in which necessary schemas are not available to guide problem solving) but is reversed for trainees with extensive prior knowledge.[51] In the latter case, more advanced or knowledgable trainees seem to perform as well or better when they are able to construct their own problems and solve them.

Related to this, there is also evidence indicating that when learners are required to generate an organization of the examples provided in learning, transfer of learning is enhanced.[52] Some have explained this finding by arguing that trainee-generated organization of examples may be more decontextualized than instructor-provided examples,[53] leading to more adaptive performance. Hence, the process of identifying the relationship among examples—which necessitates a deeper consideration of their features—seems to contribute to learning.

Scaffolding

Another strategy that has received attention in the literature is the notion that a simulated learning environment must incorporate appropriate scaffolds for learners as a means to guide them through the learning process. Bransford and colleagues[54] use the analogy of "training wheels" as a means to explain how scaffolds can be used to support the learning of tasks that students would otherwise be unable to accomplish. According to Puntambekar and Hübscher,[55] instructional scaffolds (which include hints, cues, and explanations) enable novices to solve a problem or accomplish a task that they would not otherwise be able to complete on their own. Further, many researchers assert that an important feature of scaffolds is fading, that is, removing the support so that the learner can take control. This action is essential so that the trainees eventually learn to perform the task without the aid of the scaffold, and do not become overly dependent on it.

Several methods and mechanisms for incorporating scaffolding in learning environments have been proposed, including conceptual, metacognitive, procedural, and strategic scaffolds.[56] These scaffolds can guide learners through complex tasks by directing attention during performance and providing specific directions. Moreover, in computer-based or simulation-based systems, scaffolds can take graphic form or include explicit representations of tacit aspects of the task. A classic scaffold used in aviation training is the "tunnel in the sky" used in flight simulators. Essentially, the novice pilot learns to fly from checkpoint to checkpoint by keeping his or her aircraft inside the image of a tunnel that is imposed on the visual system. With practice, the tunnel is faded so that the learner eventually learns to keep the plane steady and level.

Along these lines, Singer and Howey[57] recently described an approach to scaffolding that involves augmenting simulated environments by manipulating deviations from fidelity (ie, how close they represent the actual task situation) as a means to improve learning. By using specific cueing strategies, provisions can be added to simulations that better support the learner by ensuring that necessary exposure to, and practice with, important cues. For example, enhancing the salience of a cue in the environment through visual manipulation (eg, increased brightness, color) can help to direct the learner's attention so that he or she appropriately confronts the stimulus.

Using a somewhat different approach, Cuevas and colleagues[58] demonstrated a positive impact of scaffolding (in the form of diagrams) on cognitive and metacognitive processes in learning. In addition, adaptive scaffolding, which changes in accordance with the learner's level of mastery, has been shown to improve students' ability to self-regulate.[59] In fact, in simulation-based training, there are vast opportunities to scaffold learner performance, particularly those that are adaptive so that they change and fade over time. In particular, graphically based scaffolds are a natural choice in simulations because they can be embedded easily and unobtrusively.

Guidelines for Learning/Instructional Strategies

1. In complex scenarios, provide an introductory presentation to explain the goals of training and to direct the trainee's attention to the most important stimuli.
2. Attentional advice can be delivered in a manner similar to real-life briefings, reinforcing good teamwork skills while also augmenting training.
3. Prior to training, novice learners should be provided with a brief description of new material to be learned. This description should describe the relationships among newly introduced constructs.
4. Complex information can be presented via illustrations prior to training. This might be useful when the learner is asked to integrate disparate areas of knowledge (eg, technology and physiologic systems).
5. Early in learning, use examples (particularly worked-out examples) to demonstrate correct performance to trainees.
6. Later in training, allow trainees to explore the learning environment and develop their own examples of important lessons.
7. Develop scaffolds for novices so that they can complete more advanced tasks.
8. Use technology (ie, within the simulation) to provide hints, cues, and other scaffolds to direct the learner's attention.
9. Fade the use of scaffolds as the learner advances.

GOAL SETTING AND GOAL ORIENTATION

Goal-setting theory holds that specific, challenging (but achievable) goals are associated with the highest performance outcomes as compared with situations whereby people have no goals or are told just to do their best.[60] It has been estimated that more than 1000 studies of goal setting and its influence on performance have been conducted.[60] This body of work has identified several variables that are associated with goal setting, including choice, effort, persistence, and strategy, which appear to be the mechanisms by which goals positively affect performance. In addition, ability, commitment to the goal, feedback, and task complexity all appear to moderate the goal-performance relationship.

The one case in which specific, high goals do not appear beneficial is early in learning when this type of goal seems to overwhelm novice learners.[61] In fact, goal setting in the learning environment seems to be more complex than in other situations. For example, Dweck[62] proposed a personality trait that has been theorized to drive a trainee's personal goals for training, which has a direct impact on the eventual outcomes they achieve. Further, there are 3 specific goal-orientation states that are thought to influence training.[63] The first of these is a *mastery* orientation (sometimes called a *learning* orientation). This perspective emphasizes the acquisition of specific skills and abilities. Alternatively, a *performance-prove* orientation focuses on demonstrating one's competence, regardless of whether skill acquisition occurs or not. Finally, there is the *performance-avoid* orientation. Persons with this orientation are focused on acting in such a manner that they are not perceived as incompetent or failing. It is generally accepted that a mastery orientation leads to higher levels of intrinsic motivation than the other types.[64] In addition to increased motivation to learn, learners with a mastery orientation also seem more resilient to the challenges they encounter during training.[65]

The literature on goal orientation might be of particular importance to medical educators, especially early in students' careers. Some researchers have suggested that the culture of medical education is such that it engenders a performance-avoid orientation. That is, students believe that the important thing is to not look incompetent. The orientation of students also seems to influence the type of feedback they elicit from their instructors. Trainees with a mastery orientation seem more likely to request feedback about how to improve, whereas those with a performance orientation typically seek only validation information.[66] Not surprisingly, then, medical students with a mastery orientation are more likely to focus on the benefits of feedback, whereas students with a performance orientation are more likely to perceive feedback as a process that only exerts a toll on the learner.[67]

Given the apparent importance of the mastery orientation on training effectiveness, researchers have attempted to create interventions that result in higher levels of mastery orientation in trainees. For example, Martocchio[68] was able to induce a mastery orientation by manipulating trainees' belief about their abilities along with some instruction about how best to practice. Specifically, trainees were led to believe that increased effort could improve their abilities (as opposed to being a fixed entity) and were instructed to learn from their mistakes (as opposed to doing their best). This simple induction led to better performance and lower anxiety.

Others have been able to induce a mastery orientation through instructions given to trainees at the onset of training.[69] Still others have focused on behavioral modeling (ie, watching performers demonstrating behaviors consistent with one or another orientation) to induce desired orientations.[70] Each of these induction techniques seems effective in creating greater levels of training motivation. Goal orientation can be created through induction, which has led researchers to conclude that it may be best considered a trait (ie, more enduring personality trait) and a state (ie, situational-induced condition). In fact, according to Latham and Locke,[71] it is likely that these 2 aspects of goal orientation can interact to affect learning outcomes. These researchers reviewed several studies and concluded that setting specific, high learning goals leads to better training outcomes than setting performance goals (either specific or vague), particularly when learners are novices, and that this relationship was higher for those who were high in trait-learning orientation. Moreover, it seems that learning goals effectively shifts the trainees' attention to focus on the discovery of the strategies, processes, or procedures necessary to perform a task effectively.[71]

Researchers have also recently investigated the relationship between goal orientation and the ability of trainees to demonstrate adaptive performance after training. Obviously this is a critical area of concern for surgical training. For example, Kozlowski and colleagues[38] have recently demonstrated that a mastery orientation induction improved self-efficacy (ie, a person's belief that he or she has the requisite skills to accomplish the task) during training and was related to later adaptability. More recently, Bell and Kozlowski[72] demonstrated that a mastery induction, combined with an exploratory learning induction, leads to positive outcomes for adaptive performance.

Guidelines for Goal Setting and Orientation

1. Training material should be designed to reinforce the importance of mastery versus performance.
2. Descriptions of training and its goals as well as the content of training itself should emphasize learning rather than performance.
3. Feedback should be designed to emphasize mastery of the material rather than demonstrated performance.
4. When available, trainees should observe models performing with a mastery orientation.
5. When part of a larger curriculum, the overall training program should emphasize mastery and life-long learning.

PERFORMANCE MEASUREMENT

As observed by Issenberg and colleagues,[1] one of the essential features of a learning environment is the existence of clear benchmarks and outcomes; this implies that training performance is recorded and measured. Understanding how close a trainee's performance is to criteria is obviously essential, not only to conclude that sufficient learning has occurred but also to allow for feedback when deficiencies exist. Therefore, performance measurement and feedback are highly coupled.

In general, measuring performance is challenging in high-performance environments because it is difficult to assess complex, and often unobservable, skills. This holds true for several reasons. First, in many cases the situation is unfolding rapidly and there are many things going on at once (this is particularly true in team-level simulations). Therefore, simply tracking and sorting through trainees' performance is challenging.

Further, evaluating performance is difficult in many cases because it is impossible to track a trainee's thought process. Hence, instructors may not be able to comment on the process that the trainee used to arrive at a conclusion or action. Moreover, establishing standards of performance—a set of criteria that describe desired performance—is often not feasible in complex situations where there are many possible ways to solve a problem or targeted performance is difficult to characterize (eg, when assessing competencies such as interpersonal skills). Therefore, in many environments, accurate performance assessment requires direct observation by an instructor or coach.

In more sophisticated systems, efforts to develop computer-based expert performance models as a basis for performance measurement are beginning to gain traction. Embedded into the instructional system, expert models provide a basis for the real-time comparison of current student performance (which is recorded and organized into dynamic student models) with what would be expected by an expert in a similar situation. Gott and Lesgold[73] emphasize that this ability is enhanced when progressively sophisticated models of the expert (ie, that describe not only ultimate performance but important stages or way points in learning) are used.

Perhaps the most important function of performance measurement is the ability to diagnose the causes of observed performance. That is, it is not sufficient to say that a trainee performed poorly without understanding the causes of observed deficiencies, because interventions designed to improve performance must be based on an understanding of why the effective or ineffective behavior was demonstrated. For example, if the learner's performance can be attributed to a lack of fundamental knowledge in a basic science domain, this would suggest one remediation strategy, whereas a deficiency in skills (eg, communication, psychomotor) would suggest an entirely different one.

Over the past few decades, volumes have been written about performance measurement in general, and more specifically, how it is best accomplished in training situations. Some general conclusions from this work (particularly related to simulation-based training) include that performance measures must be tightly coupled with targeted learning objectives; that effective measures allow for comparison with an established standard of performance; and that measures must provide for a diagnosis of the causes of effective and ineffective behavior.[33] Beyond these conclusions, more specific prescriptions are expressed in the guidelines offered below.

Guidelines for Performance Measurement

1. Develop recording systems that allow instructors easy access to important performance data throughout a scenario or exercise.
2. Develop multiple measures (if possible) for all learning objectives.
3. Develop measures that allow for comparison to an established standard or metric (which also may need to be developed if they do not exist).
4. Develop expert models of performance where feasible.
5. Concentrate on developing measures that provide diagnostic information.
6. If human assessors are used, train them to avoid rating errors.

PRETRAINING MOTIVATION AND EXPECTATIONS

A final set of guidelines we highlight is related to events that occur before the learner enters the formal training environment. It seems obvious that training does not occur in a "vacuum." Rather, trainees arrive at the training experience with a wide variety of beliefs, expectations, and levels of motivation. Each of these may affect the degree to which the eventual training is effective.[74] Consequently, it is wise to attempt to optimize these pretraining factors to obtain the best possible training results. In the following sections, we briefly review the literature related to the most critical pretraining factors and provide some guidelines about interventions that allow the training profession to leverage these factors.

Pretraining Motivation

Training motivation is thought of as the intention to invest effort to engage with the training experience.[75] This is typically assessed before training begins (ie, pretraining motivation). In general, it is well established that pretraining motivation is predictive of training outcomes.[76] For example, Facteau and colleagues[77] report that the correlation between these attitudes and training outcomes was a relatively large 0.45. In an effort to better understand training motivation, psychologists have studied various factors that are thought to affect it. Many of these factors are relevant only in industrial settings and are not discussed here (the reader is directed to Colquitt and colleagues[78] for a thorough review). However, there are a few training motivation considerations that are likely to be relevant to surgical training; these are reviewed here.

Perhaps the most well understood effect of training motivation is related to the decision to participate in training. For example, Tharenou[79] conducted a large-scale questionnaire study designed to investigate the motivation-training relationship. She concluded that training motivation was an important predictor of the level of participation in training for the following year.

Another important motivational effect is related to the trainee's belief that the training will actually be useful in his or her daily work. The belief that training will have this type of use has been related to both satisfaction with training[80] and subsequent learning and transfer of training.[81,82] Although the utility of surgical simulations is likely apparent to trainees, this might be an issue when simulations are used to teach softer skills, such as communication or teamwork.[83] In this case, the importance of the information to be conveyed in training should be communicated to optimize trainee motivation.

Finally, it has been pointed out that the perceived utility of training can be underestimated if trainees overestimate their own abilities. In this case, they may perceive that their abilities cannot be improved, reducing the perceived utility and any training approach. In such cases, it may be necessary to present overconfident trainees with very difficult problems that are likely to exceed their abilities. Demonstrating that they have vulnerabilities is an effective mechanism to increase the learner's willingness to engage in training.

Expectations for Training

One specific type of pretraining motivational factor is the trainee's expectations about training. It has been argued that training fulfillment—the degree to which the actual content of training matches or exceeds the trainee's expectations—might be an important predictor of ultimate training performance.[84] There are some empirical data that support this contention. For example, Hoiberg and colleagues[85] observed the importance of trainee expectations in their study of military recruit training. Trainees who expected greater degrees of personal control and more innovations in training were more likely to be discharged without successful completion of the program. Furthermore, retrospective analyses of training fulfillment indicated that the degree to which training expectations were not meant was an important predictor of training failure.

Cannon-Bowers and colleagues[86] developed a theoretical model to predict the role of various factors on training effectiveness. Based on this research, the investigators included trainee expectations in their model. In their subsequent test of the model with navy recruits, Cannon-Bowers and colleagues found that trainee expectations were, indeed, a significant predictor of many training outcomes, including self-efficacy, trainee reactions, and physical performance.

Given the apparent importance of accurate trainee expectations, one might wonder if it is possible to intervene to increase expectation accuracy. Researchers have explored this question experimentally. For example, Hicks and Klimoski[87] attempted to improve trainee expectations through pretraining notifications. Specifically, they compared detailed, realistic descriptions of training to brief, overly optimistic descriptions. The study found that trainees who received the realistic message reported higher levels of motivation to learn and a higher degree of commitment to the training. Similar results were reported by Magjuka and Baldwin,[88] who found that trainees who obtained more information about training were eventually more satisfied with their training experience. Tai[89] also found that information from supervisors can improve trainee expectations. He reports that properly framed information about training leads to improved self-efficacy and training outcomes.

The advent of technology-based training has led researchers to consider the implications for trainee expectations. Some have suggested that the coolness factor of these technologies may lead this type of training to exceed trainee expectations, leading to positive training outcomes.[33] However, as trainees become more familiar with game and simulation technologies, they may well begin to develop expectations that are not met by the technology; this may eventually lead to unfulfilled expectations and, consequently, poor training outcomes.[90] However, there has been no empirical investigation of either effect.

Guidelines for Pretraining Motivation

1. The relationship between the skills to be trained and job performance should be articulated before training begins.
2. Trainees should be provided with objective feedback about their performance prior to training, with specific data about how the training might help them improve.
3. The importance of nontechnical skills emphasized in training should be clearly articulated before training begins.
4. Trainees should be provided with a concise, honest description of the training that they will receive.
5. Descriptions of the technology (including screenshots) might be useful in assisting trainees in creating realistic expectations.
6. When appropriate, supervisors should provide a realistic preview of the training with their subordinates.

SUMMARY AND FUTURE DIRECTIONS

Our contention throughout this article has been that simulation-based surgical education has now matured to the point at which researchers and practitioners can begin to consider instructional design features that optimize the simulation experience. This approach has the potential to improve the cost effectiveness of simulation-based training because the investment in training resources can be increased with attention to design features such as those discussed here. All of that said, we believe that there are several research needs that warrant further attention.

First of all, there is a need for more longitudinal studies so that the long-term impact of these features on learning and retention can be addressed more fully. Throughout the training literature there are far too few such studies—surgery has the potential to lead in this crucial area. Related to this is the investigation of training transfer, which is affected by many variables (besides time). If training interventions are to be truly validated, rigorous investigations of how performance changes in the actual work environment are essential. It will not be possible to address return on investment issues until such data are collected.

We would also like to see investigation of hybrid models of practice and feedback that begin with part-task training, shorter practice intervals, and frequent feedback but then move to the whole-task, longer practice intervals and less frequent feedback. Such studies are needed, particularly in simulation-based environments and with tasks that have complex performance requirements. Another useful approach would be to assess the differential impact of simulation-based training on different surgical competencies and how best to structure practice, feedback, and learning strategies for different competencies within the simulation environment. Finally, we hope that researchers will consider including personality factors when studying simulation-based surgical training. We have made a case for trait goal orientation; other variables such as self-efficacy (which has been shown definitively to have an impact on learning, transfer, and performance) should be considered as well.[90]

Regarding the future of simulation-based surgical research, we are encouraged by all the good work that has already been done and prospects for the future. Simulation offers tremendous (unparalleled) opportunities to improve the preparation of surgeons and, in turn, patient outcomes. Moreover, technological advances are making even highly complex, virtual environments cost effective and feasible in all phases of surgical education. We are just beginning to scratch the surface of these opportunities, and look forward to a flood of well-designed, scientifically rigorous studies that enable us to optimize their implementation. We are also encouraged because surgical simulation seems to have stimulated applied training research in the same way that the aviation industry did in the 1990s. A side benefit of this phenomenon is that our knowledge of training for all types of tasks improves as a function of focusing on surgical competencies. The result is that the general training literature evolves and matures for all types of learning situations.

REFERENCES

1. Issenberg SB, McGaghie WC, Petrusa ER, et al. Features and uses of high-fidelity medical simulations that lead to effective learning: a BEME systematic review. Med Teacher 2005;27(1):10–28.
2. Russell JD. Book review: principles of instructional design, 5th edition. Perform Improv 2007;44(2):44–6.
3. Reiser RA, Gagne RM. Characteristics of media selection models. Rev Educ Res 1982;52(4):499–512.
4. Hewson M, Little M. Giving feedback in medical education: verification of recommended techniques. J Gen Intern Med 1998;13(2):111–6.
5. Bangert-Drowns RL, Kulik CC, Kulik JA, et al. The instructional effect of feedback in test-like events. Rev Educ Res 1991;61(2):213–38.
6. Earley PC, Northcraft GB, Lee C, et al. Impact of process and outcome feedback on the relation of goal setting to task performance. Acad Manage J 1990;33(1):87–105.
7. Balzer WK, Doherty ME, O'Connor R. Effects of cognitive feedback on performance. Psychol Bull 1989;106(3):410–33.
8. Korsgaard MA, Diddams M. The effect of process feedback and task complexity on personal goals, information searching, and performance improvement. J Appl Soc Psychol 1996;26(21):1889–911.
9. Anderson JR, Corbett AT, Koedinger KR, et al. Cognitive tutors: lessons learned. J Learn Sci 1995;4(2):167–207.
10. Gibson FP. Feedback delays: how can decision makers learn not to buy a new car every time the garage is empty? Organ Behav Hum Decis Process 2000;83(1):141–66.
11. Schmidt RA, Bjork RA. New conceptualizations of practice: common principles in three paradigms suggest new concepts for training. Psychol Sci 1992;3(4):207–17.
12. Kulik JA, Kulik CC. Timing of feedback and verbal learning. Rev Educ Res 1988;58(1):79–97.
13. Schooler LJ, Anderson JR. The role of process in the rational analysis of memory. Cognit Psychol 1997;32(3):219–50.
14. Scroth M. The effects of delay of feedback on a delayed concept formation transfer task. Contemp Educ Psychol 1992;17(1):78–82.
15. Xeroulis G, Park J, Moulton C, et al. Teaching suturing and knot-tying skills to medical students: a randomized controlled study comparing computer-based

video instruction and (concurrent and summary) expert feedback. Surgery 2007; 141(4):442–9.

16. Walsh C, Ling S, Wang C, et al. Concurrent versus terminal feedback: it may be better to wait. Acad Med 2009;84(10):S54–7.

17. McLaughlin A, Rogers W. Fisk A. Feedback support for training: accounting for learner and task. In: Proceedings of the Human Factors and Ergonomics Society 52nd Annual Meeting, September 22–6, 2008. New York (NY): Human Factors and Ergonomics Society; 2008. p. 2624–8.

18. Schmidt RA, Young DE, Swinnen S, et al. Summary knowledge of results for skill acquisition: support for the guidance hypothesis. J Exp Psychol Learn Mem Cogn 1989;15(2):352–9.

19. Wickens C. Multiple resources and performance prediction. In: Moray N, editor. Ergonomics: psychological mechanisms and models in ergonomics. New York: Taylor & Francis; 2005. p. 83–105.

20. van Merriënboer J, Clark R, de Croock M. Blueprints for complex learning: the 4c/id-model. Educ Tech Res Dev 2002;50(2):39–64.

21. Lim J, Reiser RA. Effects of part-task and whole-task instructional approaches and levels of learner expertise on learner acquisition and transfer of a complex cognitive skill. International Conference on Learning Sciences. In: Proceedings of the 7th International Conference on Learning Sciences, June 27 to July 1, 2006. Bloomington (IN): International Society of the Learning Sciences; 2006. p. 425–31.

22. Naylor JC, Briggs GE. Effect of rehearsal of temporal and spatial aspects on the long-term retention of a procedural skill. J Appl Psychol 1963;47(2):120–6.

23. Mattoon J. Learner control and part/whole-task practice methods in instructional simulation. San Antonio (TX): Amstriong Air Force Base Technical Report; 1992.

24. van Merriënboer JJ, Sweller J. Cognitive load theory and complex learning: recent developments and future directions. Educ Psychol Rev 2005;17(2): 147–77.

25. Paas FG, Van Merriënboer JJ. Instructional control of cognitive load in the training of complex cognitive tasks. Educ Psychol Rev 1994;6(4):351–71.

26. Son LK. Spacing one's study: evidence for a metacognitive control strategy. J Exp Psychol Learn Mem Cogn 2004;30(3):601–9.

27. Cepeda NJ, Coburn N, Rohrer D, et al. Optimizing distributed practice: theoretical analysis and practical implications. Exp Psychol 2009;56(4):236–46.

28. Pashler H, Rohrer D, Cepeda NJ, et al. Enhancing learning and retarding forgetting: choices and consequences. Psychon Bull Rev 2007;14(2):187–93.

29. Cepeda NJ, Pashler H, Vul E, et al. Distributed practice in verbal recall tasks: a review and quantitative synthesis. Psychol Bull 2006;132(3):354–80.

30. Glenberg AM, Lehmann TS. Spacing repetitions over 1 week. Mem Cognit 1980; 8(6):528–38.

31. Bahrick HP, Bahrick LE, Bahrick AS, et al. Maintenance of foreign language vocabulary and the spacing effect. Psychol Sci 1993;4(5):316–21.

32. Salas E, Rhodenizer L, Bowers CA. The design and delivery of crew resource management training: exploiting available resources. Hum Factors 2000;42(3): 490–511 Publisher:US: Human Factors & Ergonomics Society.

33. Cannon-Bowers J, Bowers C. Synthetic learning environments: on developing a science of simulation, games, and virtual worlds for training. In: Kozlowski SW, Salas E, editors. Learning, training, and development in organizations. New York (NY): Routledge; 2010 p. 229–61.

34. Cannon-Bowers JA. Recent advances in scenario-based training for medical education. Curr Opin Anaesthesiol 2008;21(6):784–9.

35. Oser RL, Cannon-Bowers JA, Salas E, et al. Enhancing human performance in technology-rich environments: guidelines for scenario-based training. Human/Technology Interaction in Complex Systems 1999;9:175–202.
36. Dwyer DJ, Fowlkes JE, Oser RL, et al. Team performance measurement in distributed environments: the TARGETs methodology. In: Brannick MT, editor. Team performance assessment and measurement: theory, methods, and applications. Mahwah (NJ): Lawrence Erlbaum; 1997. p. 137–53.
37. Fowlkes J, Dwyer DJ, Oser RL, et al. Event-based approach to training (EBAT). Int J Aviat Psychol 1998;8(3):209–21.
38. Kozlowski SW, Gully SM, Brown KG, et al. Effects of training goals and goal orientation traits on multidimensional training outcomes and performance adaptability. Organ Behav Hum Decis Process 2001;85(1):1–31.
39. Mayer RE, Moreno R. Nine ways to reduce cognitive load in multimedia learning. Educ Psychol 2003;38(1):43–52.
40. Sweller J. Cognitive load theory, learning difficulty, and instructional design. Learn Instruct 1994;4(4):295–312.
41. Lee H, Plass JL, Homer BD. Optimizing cognitive load for learning from computer-based science simulations. J Educ Psychol 2006;98(4):902–13.
42. Cannon-Bowers JA, Rhodenizer L, Salas E, et al. A framework for understanding pre-practice conditions and their impact on learning. Person Psychol 1998;51(2):291–320.
43. Phye GD. Schemata training and transfer of an intellectual skill. J Educ Psychol 1989;81(3):347–52.
44. Ausubel D. Educational psychology: a cognitive view. New York: Holt, Rinehart and Winston; 1968.
45. Preiss RW, Gayle BM. A meta-analysis of the educational benefits of employing advanced organizers. In: Gayle BM, Preiss RW, Burrell N, editors. Classroom communication and instructional processes: advances through meta-analysis. Mahwah (NJ): Lawerence Erlbaum; 2006. p. 329–44.
46. Paivio A, Clark JM. The role of topic and vehicle imagery in metaphor comprehension. Communication and Cognition 1986;19(3–4):367–87.
47. Quealy J, Langan-Fox J. Attributes of delivery media in computer-assisted instruction. Ergonomics 1998;41(3):257–79.
48. Anderson JR, Schunn CD. Implications of the ACT-R learning theory: no magic bullets. In: Glaser R, editor. Advances in instructional psychology: educational design and cognitive science, 5. Mahwah (NJ): Lawrence Erlbaum; 2000. p. 1–34.
49. Sweller J, van Merrienboer JJ, Paas FG. Cognitive architecture and instructional design. Educ Psychol Rev 1998;10(3):251–96.
50. Sweller J. Discussion of 'emerging topics in cognitive load research: using learner and information characteristics in the design of powerful learning environments'. Appl Cogn Psychol 2006;20(3):353–7.
51. Kalyuga S, Chandler P, Tuovinen J, et al. When problem solving is superior to studying worked examples. J Educ Psychol 2001;93(3):579–88.
52. di Vesta FJ, Peverly ST. The effects of encoding variability, processing activity, and rule—examples sequence on the transfer of conceptual rules. J Educ Psychol 1984;76(1):108–19.
53. Clark RE, Voogel A. Transfer of training principles for instructional design. Educ Comm Tech J 1985;33(2):113–23.
54. Bransford JD, Brown AL, Cocking RR. How people learn: brain, mind, experience, and school. Washington, DC: US: National Academy Press; 1999.

55. Puntambekar S, Hübscher R. Tools for scaffolding students in a complex learning environment: what have we gained and what have we missed? Educ Psychol 2005;40(1):1–12.

56. Hannafin M, Land S, Oliver K. Open learning environments: foundation, methods, and models. In: Reigeluth CM, editor. Instructional-design theories and models: a new paradigm of instructional theory, II. Mahwah (NJ): Lawrence Erlbaum; 1999. p. 115–40.

57. Singer MJ, Howey AM. Enhancing virtual environments to support training. In: Schmarrow D, Cohn J, Nicholson DM, editors. The PSI handbook of virtual environments for training and education: developments for the military and beyond, vols. 1–3. Westport (CT): Praeger; 2008. p. 407–21.

58. Cuevas HM, Fiore SM, Oser RL. Scaffolding cognitive and metacognitive processes in low verbal ability learners: use of diagrams in computer-based training environments. Instructional Science 2002;30(6):433–64.

59. Azevedo R, Cromley JG, Winters FI, et al. Adaptive human scaffolding facilitates adolescents' self-regulated learning with hypermedia. Instructional Science 2005; 33(5–6):381–412.

60. Locke E, Latham G. Building a practically useful theory of goal setting and task motivation: a 35-year odyssey. Am Psychol 2002;57(9):705–17.

61. Kanfer R, Ackerman P. Dynamics of skill acquisition: building a bridge between intelligence and motivation. In: Sternberg RJ, editor, Advances in the psychology of human intelligence, vol. 5. Mahwah (NJ): Lawrence Erlbaum Associates, Inc; 1989. p. 83–134 [e-book].

62. Dweck CS. Motivational processes affecting learning. American Psychologist 1986;41(10):1040–8 Special issue: psychological science and education.

63. Middleton MJ, Midgley C. Avoiding the demonstration of lack of ability: an under-explored aspect of goal theory. J Educ Psychol 1997;89(4):710–8.

64. Rawsthorne LJ, Elliott AJ. Achievement goals and intrinsic motivation: a meta-analytic review. Pers Soc Psychol Rev 1999;3(4):326–44.

65. Colquitt JA, Simmering MJ. Conscientiousness, goal orientation, and motivation to learn during the learning process: a longitudinal study. J Appl Psychol 1998; 83(4):654–65.

66. Janssen O, Prins J. Goal orientations and the seeking of different types of feedback information. J Occup Organ Psychol 2007;80(2):235–49.

67. Teunissen PW, Stapel DA, Scheele F, et al. The influence of context on residents' evaluations: effects of priming on clinical judgment and affect. Adv Health Sci Educ Theory Pract 2009;14(1):23–41.

68. Martocchio JJ. Effects of conceptions of ability on anxiety, self-efficacy, and learning in training. J Appl Psychol 1994;79(6):819–25.

69. Winters D, Latham GP. The effect of learning versus outcome goals on a simple versus a complex task. Group Organ Manag 1996;21(2):236–50.

70. Gist ME, Stevens CK. Effects of practice conditions and supplemental training method on cognitive learning and interpersonal skill generalization. Organ Behav Hum Decis Process 1998;75(2):142–69.

71. Latham G, Locke E. New developments in and directions for goal-setting research. Eur Psychol 2007;12(4):290–300.

72. Bell BS, Kozlowski SW. Active learning: effects of core training design elements on self-regulatory processes, learning, and adaptability. J Appl Psychol 2008; 93(2):296–316.

73. Gott SP, Lesgold AM. Competence in the workplace: How cognitive performance models and situated instruction can accelerate skill acquisition. In:

Glaser R, editor. Advances in instructional psychology: educational design and cognitive science, vol. 5. Mahwah (NJ): Lawrence Erlbaum; 2000. p. 239–328.

74. Noe RA. Trainees' attributes and attitudes: neglected influences on training effectiveness. Acad Manage Rev 1986;11(4):736–49.

75. Tannenbaum SI, Yukl G. Training and development in work organizations. Annu Rev Psychol 1992;43:399–441.

76. Burke LA, Hutchins HM. A study of best practices in training transfer and proposed model of transfer. Hum Resource Dev Q 2008;19(2):107–28.

77. Facteau JD, Dobbins GH, Russell JE, et al. The influence of general perceptions of the training environment on pretraining motivation and perceived training transfer. J Manag 1995;21(1):1–25.

78. Colquitt JA, LePine JA, Noe RA. Toward an integrative theory of training motivation: a meta-analytic path analysis of 20 years of research. J Appl Psychol 2000; 85(5):678–707.

79. Tharenou P. The relationship of training motivation to participation in training and development. J Occup Organ Psychol 2001;74(5):599–621.

80. Clark CS, Dobbins GH, Ladd RT. Exploratory field study of training motivation: influence of involvement, credibility, and transfer climate. Group Organ Manag 1993;18(3):292–307.

81. Baumgartel HJ, Reynolds JI, Pathan RZ. How personality and organisational climate variables moderate the effectiveness of management development programmes: a review and some recent research findings. Management and Labour Studies 1984;9(1):1–16.

82. Lim DH, Morris ML. Influence of trainee characteristics, instructional satisfaction, and organizational climate on perceived learning and training transfer. Hum Resource Dev Q 2006;17(1):85–115.

83. Yedidia MJ, Lipkin M, Schwartz MD, et al. Doctors as workers: work-hour regulations and interns' perceptions of responsibility, quality of care, and training. J Gen Intern Med 1993;8(8):429–35.

84. Tannenbaum SI, Mathieu JE, Salas E, et al. Meeting trainees' expectations: the influence of training fulfillment on the development of commitment, self-efficacy, and motivation. J Appl Psychol 1991;76(6):759–69.

85. Hoiberg A, Booth RF, Berry NH. Non-cognitive variables related to performance in Navy 'A' schools. Psychol Rep 1977;41(2):647–55.

86. Cannon-Bowers JA, Salas E, Tannenbaum SI, et al. Toward theoretically based principles of training effectiveness: a model and initial empirical investigation. Mil Psychol 1995;7(3):141–64.

87. Hicks WD, Klimoski RJ. Entry into training programs and its effects on training outcomes: a field experiment. Acad Manage J 1987;30(3):542–52.

88. Magjuka RJ, Baldwin TT. Team-based employee involvement programs: effects of design and administration. Personnel Psychology 1991;44(4): 793–812.

89. Tai W. Effects of training framing, general self-efficacy and training motivation on trainees' training effectiveness. Person Rev 2006;35(1):51–65.

90. Bandura A. Self-efficacy: the foundation of agency. In: Perrig WJ, Grobb A, editor. Control of human behavior, mental processes, and consciousness: essays in honor of the 60th birthday of August Flammer. Mahwah (NJ): Lawrence Erlbaum; 2000. p. 17–33.

Virtual Reality in Surgical Skills Training

Vanessa N. Palter, MD[a],*, Teodor P. Grantcharov, MD, PhD[b]

KEYWORDS

- Simulation • Virtual reality • Technical skills • Assessment
- Nontechnical skills • Curriculum development

The traditional system of surgical training as outlined by Halstead more than a century ago has been challenged by numerous recent developments. These developments include a decrease in resident work hours, a decrease in available operating-room time, an ethical imperative to protect patients from harm, and a unique skill set required for endoscopic techniques and minimally invasive surgery.[1–3] It is now widely accepted that some degree of technical skills training outside the operating room (OR) is imperative for surgical residents.[4]

Virtual reality (VR) offers enormous potential to enhance technical skills training outside the operating room. Training on a virtual-reality system avoids the ethical concerns associated with practice on animals or cadavers. In addition, virtual-reality simulation allows for a more flexible environment than can be created by low- and high-fidelity bench-top models. Many of the current VR systems allow for practice at varying levels of difficulty and across a wide range of clinical scenarios, thus accommodating learners at many levels. VR also allows for repeated practice without any risk to patients. Finally, virtual reality has the potential for formative and summative assessment because of the fact that these simulators can provide standardized conditions and generate automatic assessment measures.[5]

Although the potential of VR simulators in surgical education is widely acknowledged, a significant challenge for educators is deciding, among the many VR simulators available, which is ideal for implementation in their particular program. It is necessary to not only choose a simulator that has demonstrated acceptable validity in the literature but also to determine a schedule for training on the simulator, determine appropriate assessment parameters, and define expert competencies. This article reviews the role of virtual reality in a curriculum for the teaching and assessment

[a] The Wilson Centre, Toronto General Hospital, 200 Elizabeth Street, Room 1ES-565, Toronto, ON M5G 2C4, Canada
[b] Department of Surgery, St Michael's Hospital, University of Toronto, Room 16CC-056, 30 Bond Street, Toronto, ON M5W 1W8, Canada
* Corresponding author.
E-mail address: vanessa.palter@utoronto.ca

Surg Clin N Am 90 (2010) 605–617
doi:10.1016/j.suc.2010.02.005
0039-6109/10/$ – see front matter
surgical.theclinics.com

of technical skills. The evidence regarding the role of VR in learning technical skills is examined and elements necessary for effective curriculum design are explored.

LEARNING TECHNICAL SKILLS ON VIRTUAL-REALITY SYSTEMS

The technical skills required to perform laparoscopic surgery and endoscopy differ substantially from those required for open surgical procedures. Indeed, a requirement of performing endoscopic or laparoscopic procedures is watching a two-dimensional video on a screen, becoming accustomed to limited tactile feedback and to the fulcrum effect of working with long instruments.[6] Training on virtual-reality models before practice in the operating room allows for the concept of a "pre-trained novice" whereby trainees overcome the early phase of their learning curve in a simulated environment, thus contributing to their learning efficiency in the operating room.[7,8]

Learning has been shown on a variety of virtual-reality systems, including those designed to teach bronchoscopy, colonoscopy, gastroscopy, minimally invasive surgery, and specific urological techniques. Learning curves of the Minimally Invasive Surgical Trainer-Virtual Reality (MIST-VR), a low fidelity VR simulator designed to teach the technical skill set for laparoscopic surgery, are perhaps the most well defined in the literature. Studies have shown that novices reach expert proficiency after approximately 10 trials on the simulator[9] and that learning curves exhibit individual variations.[10,11] This finding is important because it indicates that trainees at similar levels may take different amounts of time to reach expert proficiency. After proficiency has been achieved, some degree of retention of what was learned persisted after 7 months.[12] In addition, learning curves on different laparoscopic VR systems have been shown to be comparable, with experts plateauing first, and intermediates and novices exhibiting a longer learning curve.[13-15]

The learning curves that have been defined for VR simulators for laparoscopy are similar to those described for bronchoscopic, urologic, and endoscopic VR simulators.[16-21] It can be difficult to make comparisons across studies because duration of training, and technical-skill evaluation methods differ between trials. However, as a group, these studies illustrate that training on VR simulators can ultimately result in novices attaining expert proficiency as measured on the simulator, and that learning eventually plateaus for novices and experts. These learning curve plateaus also reflect what has been shown on laparoscopic VR simulators where experts seem to plateau after one or two trials, whereas novices tend to plateau much later, after a minimum of six trials depending on the task in question.

This group of studies illustrates that learning on a VR simulator occurs to a greater degree with novices, and that the learning curves to attain expert proficiency differ between trainees. This finding underscores the importance of training to a level of expert proficiency as opposed to training for a certain amount of time, which is important when designing a surgical skills curriculum.

TRANSFER OF TECHNICAL SKILL FROM VIRTUAL REALITY TO THE OPERATING ROOM

The ultimate goal of learning a technical skill on a virtual-reality simulator is to increase proficiency in performance in an analogous clinical situation. As such, determining whether the skills learned on a VR simulator are transferable to the real operating room is an essential step in determining the value of a VR simulator and how best to incorporate it into a surgical skills curriculum. Although there are few well-designed, randomized, controlled trials examining skills transfer for VR simulators, these studies in general support the use of VR training to improve operative skills.

There are few studies examining skills transfer for bronchoscopy simulation. Only one small study (three subjects per group) showed improved performance in live bronchoscopy after VR training compared with a control group who received traditional training.[22] The skills learned on the VR simulator transfer to fiber-optic incubation, a live, unrelated procedure.[23] The idea that transfer of VR-acquired skills to an unrelated procedure has implications for curriculum design. Indeed, this emphasizes the fact that perhaps it is not necessary to provide training on specific VR simulators for specific technical skills, but rather that the techniques acquired on one simulator can transfer to other live, minimally invasive or endoscopic tasks. This transferability would dramatically reduce the time, cost, and expert requirements in the design of a surgical skills curriculum.

There is strong evidence for skills transfer of VR training in colonoscopy. A blinded, randomized, controlled trial by Park and colleagues[24] showed improved performance on a well-validated global assessment measure during live colonoscopy by a group that trained on a VR simulator as compared with a group that received no training. These differences persisted for the first 10 live colonoscopies.[25] Similarly, in a large, multicenter, blinded, randomized, controlled trial that assessed the effects of VR training on the first 200 colonoscopies performed by gastroenterology fellows, the VR trained group outperformed the control group, with the effect being largest for the first 40 cases performed in real subjects.[26] Although one study showed no difference in VR training as compared with conventional training, this study suffered from a small sample size and lack of blinding.[27] It can therefore be concluded that for colonoscopy, the skills learned in a virtual environment result in better performance during the initial phase of the learning curve on real patients.

For gastroscopy, the evidence for skills transfer of VR training is contradictory with some studies showing an effect and others demonstrating no significant gain from VR training. Two randomized, controlled trials demonstrate that skills learned on a gastroscopy VR simulator transfer to real patients.[28] However, a larger study by Sedlack[29] showed that skills learned on an upper-endoscopy simulator did not transfer to a clinical situation.

The transfer of skills from a virtual environment to laparoscopic procedures in the operating room has been demonstrated in several randomized trials. Seymour and colleagues[30] randomized residents to two groups: a VR group where residents trained to expert levels of proficiency and a control group. In the operating room, VR-trained residents performed a laparoscopic cholecystectomy significantly better with respect to time, a decreased injury rate, and were more likely to progress. These results were replicated by Grantcharov and colleagues[31] in a blinded, randomized, controlled study with validated assessment measures.

As a group, these studies illustrate evidence that endoscopic and laparoscopic skills learned using virtual-reality simulation will transfer to the operating room. These findings were summarized in a consensus document created by the European Association for Endoscopic Surgeons in 2005, and in a 2006 meta-analysis by Sutherland and colleagues.[32,33] Assessing the strength of the evidence for skills transfer of a simulator is essential in the design of a surgical skills curriculum. As previously stated, this allows for the idea of a pre-trained novice whereby the early learning curve inherent to many laparoscopic and endoscopic procedures is achieved in the surgical skills laboratory, thus increasing patient safety, and allowing for more effective learning by the trainee once they have the opportunity to practice and learn in a real clinical situation.

TECHNICAL SKILLS ASSESSMENT IN VIRTUAL-REALITY ENVIRONMENTS

Assessment of a trainee's technical performance on a virtual reality simulator, combined with meaningful feedback, is an essential component of the learning process.[32] Traditionally, trainees have been assessed using non-validated, unreliable tools, such as log books or subjective reports from senior colleagues. Virtual-reality simulators, however, have the ability to provide automatic, instantaneous, non-biased measures of performance.[34] This assessment can serve to monitor progress while learning a technical skill, can aid in the provision of structured feedback, and ultimately ensures that the training objectives have been met. Virtual-reality simulators, like any tool that is used for the assessment of technical skills, must demonstrate acceptable reliability and validity before they are integrated into high-stakes assessment. Reliability measures the ability of a test to produce the same results if repeated several times, whereas validity assesses whether a test in fact measures what it is designed to measure. There are various components of validity. Face validity is the degree to which a model resembles a situation in real life, construct validity measures whether the test can distinguish between different levels of experiences, concurrent validity compares the test to the gold standard, and predictive validity determines whether the test corresponds to actual performance in the operating room.[6]

The majority of studies designed to investigate the role of virtual-reality simulators as assessment devices for technical skill have focused on the demonstration of construct and face validity. In colonoscopy simulation, studies have demonstrated excellent face and construct validity of several commercially available systems.[20,22,29,35-43] However, aspects of the face validity of the upper endoscopic modules have been criticized. Experts have commented that intubation of the esophagus, which is one of the most difficult steps of the real procedure, is consistently too easy in virtual reality.[28,38,41] Face and construct validity have also been shown for many of the available urologic VR simulators.[44-49] The difficulty in interpreting results from these studies is that although they all demonstrate the ability of the simulator to distinguish between experts, intermediates and novices, the parameters that effectively differentiate these groups differs between studies. The parameters that seem to show the most evidence supporting their use in assessment are the time taken for the procedure, a measure of the amount of visualization, and a composite error score, for example "occurrence of perforations" or "time in red out."

Laparoscopic VR simulators also have shown acceptable face and construct validity, with effective discrimination between novices, intermediates, and experts.[9,14,15,50-57] As was found for endoscopic simulators, the most useful parameters for assessment in the majority of commercially available simulation systems are time, error and economy–of–movement scores. A smaller number of concurrent validation studies for minimally invasive VR simulators exist.[58,59] Kundhal and Grantcharov effectively demonstrated a correlation between VR-derived metrics with scores on the Objective Structured Assessment of Technical Skills (OSATS) global rating scale, an assessment tool that has been well validated in the literature.[58] In addition, test-retest validity has also been shown for laparoscopic VR simulators.[41]

The demonstration of construct, concurrent, and face validity across a range of virtual-reality simulators has wide implications for training programs. Performance on these simulators could be used to track progress as a trainee learns a task or to define expert levels of proficiency to determine when a trainee is ready to progress to learning in a real operating room and practice on real patients. It is important to note, however, that as a group, these studies serve to illustrate that not all assessment parameters on a VR simulator are of equal validity and that the parameters that have the most evidence to support their use are time, economy of movement, and error scores for that particular task. These three assessment parameters are useful in that they are consistent across various types of simulators. However, it is important to note that assessment is not equivalent to feedback. Indeed, these parameters generated by the simulator are not necessarily meaningful for trainees and may not provide them with insight into the weaknesses of their performance. As such, although assessment parameters are invaluable for monitoring the technical progress of trainees, they should not be used as a substitute for expert feedback.

VIRTUAL-REALITY CURRICULUM FOR TECHNICAL-SKILLS ACQUISITION

Virtual-reality training systems are effective tools for the teaching and the assessment of technical skills, however, as Seymour states, it is time to move beyond this positive data and formulate practical recommendations for the training of technical skills within a structured curriculum.[60] Several curricula for technical skills training have been described in the literature. These include a curriculum to teach laparoscopic suturing, laparoscopic cholecystectomy, and general laparoscopic skills.[4,61,62] The basic laparoscopic curriculum described by Panait and colleagues[4] consists of 17 practice modules and seven examination modules. Currently there is consensus that residents should demonstrate proficiency on a VR simulator before performing procedures in the operating room.

An effective curriculum consists of not only the opportunity to learn and be assessed on a simulator but also a system of deliberate practice and structured feedback within a specific schedule of proficiency-based training. Deliberate practice as outlined by Ericsson is essential in the creation and maintenance of expertise,[63] which refers to the idea of repetitive practice in which the desired goal continually exceeds the current level of performance.[63] Moreover, distributed practice is superior to massed practice for the learning and the retention of technical skills.[64,65] The type of practice on the simulator also affects the quality of learning. Ali and colleagues[66] demonstrated that novices practicing at a harder level on a VR simulator exhibited significantly greater learning (measured by speed, accuracy, and error) than those who practiced at an easier level. Studies have also shown that skills deteriorate without ongoing, long-term practice.[12] To address this, it has been suggested that maintenance training should be an essential part of a surgical skills curriculum, and that refresher sessions every 1 to 3 months for all the skills learned to date should be an integral part of the training schedule.[67]

In addition to deliberate practice, structured feedback is essential to learning on a virtual-reality simulator. Datta and colleagues[35] demonstrated that when no critique of performance was given during colonoscopy training, study participants did not exhibit any improvement in performance. In addition, Kruglikova and colleagues[68] showed that constructive, expert feedback resulted in faster learning on the simulator than simply relying on the automatic feedback provided by the simulator. It has also been shown that summery expert feedback, as opposed to concurrent feedback or motion efficiency feedback is more conducive to learning.[69,70] Although virtual-reality simulators have the advantage of being able to automatically generate performance assessment parameters, these studies illustrate that these automatic assessments or comments from the virtual expert should not completely replace expert feedback, which plays an essential role in learning technical skill.

When designing a technical skills curriculum, the initial step is choosing a VR simulator that is appropriate for the task. Next, one must choose a simulator with sufficient evidence of validity as a training tool. Moreover, it is essential to investigate which assessment parameters specific to that simulator have demonstrated validity in the literature. These findings are summarized in a 2006 review by Sutherland and colleagues[32,33] and a consensus document created by the European Association for Endoscopic Surgeons in 2005. Next, determining a schedule for deliberate, distributed practice and for expert summary feedback is essential to obtain maximal learning from the trainee. Finally, one must define parameters of expertise on the simulator and have trainees train to meet these levels, rather than training for specific amounts of time. Ultimately, examining the effectiveness of the curriculum and the transfer validity of the curriculum to the operating room will allow for further refinement and development of curricular goals.

THE SIMULATED OPERATING ROOM AND THE ROLE OF VIRTUAL REALITY

Although technical excellence is essential for practicing surgeons, and as such much of the virtual reality technology has focused on developing tools to effectively teach technical skills, nontechnical aspects of performance are equally essential in the creation and maintenance of surgical expertise. Previous reports have shown that many errors in the operating room are not caused by technical factors, but rather by breakdowns in nontechnical skills.[71–74] Nontechnical skills include factors, such as communication, team work, decision making, situational awareness, task management, and leadership.[74] Traditionally, the value of formal teaching and assessment of these skills in residency training programs has been under estimated, and thus, the development of nontechnical skills in trainees is done in a variable, informal, tacit manner.[74] With the large impact that the acquisition of nontechnical skills has on patient safety, and on appropriate operating room dynamics, this is no longer acceptable. To assess and teach technical and nontechnical skills, a simulated operating room designed to replicate the complexities of a real operating room has been described by various groups.[75–78] Although most of the simulated operating rooms make use of a physical simulator (mannequin) to represent patients,[75] Paige and colleagues[79] describe a simulated OR that makes use of a mannequin and a virtual-reality simulator to assess technical ability. In this study, teams consisting of nursing staff, anesthetists, and surgeons were required to manage a scenario consisting of a patient developing atrial fibrillation during a laparoscopic cholecystectomy. Technical ability was assessed on the VR simulator, while experts who observed how the individual team members interacted assessed nontechnical skills. The incorporation of virtual reality into this scenario created a more realistic environment for the assessment of technical and nontechnical skills. Indeed clinically, a surgeon must focus on their technical performance while maintaining appropriate communication with other members of the team, including the OR nurses and anesthetists. Although training in the simulated OR requires a significant time and financial commitment, this example illustrates how the incorporation of virtual reality can facilitate the training and assessment of technical and nontechnical skills in individuals across several disciplines.

VIRTUAL PATIENT SIMULATION

The development of virtual patient technology is also a medium in which technical and nontechnical skills can be assessed and taught. Screen-based VR simulation describes a situation where a trainee interacts with a computer-based simulated patient. Depending on what the trainee inputs into the system, the virtual patient responds on the screen in a predictable physiologic manner. These computer-based learning environments allow trainees to interact directly with a virtual patient and practice history taking, physical examination, and procedural skills. One of the earliest models described is CyberPatient (CyberActive Technology Ltd, Singapore) which is a software program developed in 1999 specifically for surgical trainees.[80] CyberPatient allows students to practice history taking (the virtual patient provides realistic responses depending on what questions are asked); physical examination (including the capabilities for observation, palpation, and special tests, such as sigmoidoscopy); ancillary tests; treatment planning; surgery; postoperative management; and follow-up.[80] Similar models have been developed for anesthesia and emergency medicine.[81,82] A randomized, blinded study demonstrated that screen-based patient simulation is superior to traditional training as measured by resident performance on a simulated anesthesia crisis scenario on a mannequin.[81,82] Similarly, improved history-taking skills were shown in a group of screen-based VR trained medical students in a randomized, controlled trial.[83] Although screen-based VR patient simulation seems to be a feasible, effective method of teaching surgical patient management to trainees, these VR systems have yet to be widely used in residency or training programs, and more research is required to better define their use for surgical training.

Advances in gaming simulation techniques have taken screen-based simulations a step further with the creation of virtual-reality worlds that are either Web or locally accessed. In these virtual worlds, the trainee can interact with virtual patients to investigate a clinical problem. This virtual interaction is different than screen-based simulation in that in the virtual world, the trainee sees himself or herself in the same environment as the virtual patient. These three-dimensional virtual worlds make it possible for multiple trainees, who may be located in diverse geographic locations, to take on an avatar (a virtual-reality character) in the online virtual environment.[84] Trainees can move their avatar using a mouse, can talk in real time to other players using a headset and microphone, and can initiate actions, such a using a stethoscope or a venipuncture, by choosing options from a control menu.[84] Several medical and team training scenarios have been developed for virtual worlds, including emergency room team training for the management of trauma, and team disaster-preparedness training.[85] Second Life (Linden Research, San Francisco, CA, USA) is the most popular virtual world accessible to the public.[86] Although Second Life was primarily developed for social networking, medical teaching and learning opportunities have been developed in this virtual world.[86] Players in Second Life can participate in a virtual clinic to learn about heart murmurs, learn in a virtual neurologic education center, or practice physical examinations and reading radiological films.[86,87] Although surgical-specific education modules have yet to be developed for Second Life, the potential of this technology for surgical education is vast. This environment has the potential to teach full patient-based care, including technical and nontechnical skills. More research is needed, however, to investigate the educational outcomes of engaging in a virtual world, to assess whether skills learned in a virtual world transfer to real-world patient encounters, and to define their optimal role within a surgical skills curriculum.

All the patients previously described in screen-based VR simulation, or in a virtual world, are designed to represent a certain clinical condition to teach general medical skills. For the more experienced practitioner, however, technical innovations have made it possible to practice surgical procedures based on specific patient anatomy with the goal being to develop an operative plan before performing the procedure in reality. Currently these have been described for ventriculoscopy, carotid artery stenting, excision of cerebral arteriovenous (AV) malformations, orbital and maxillofacial surgery, orthopedic procedures, and hepatic surgery.[88–93] This concept can be taken even further with the simulation of not only the anatomy of a particular patient but also their physiology to predict patient-specific effects of certain medical treatments. This concept has been described for the treatment of patients with HIV, AV malformations, and cerebral aneurysms.[94] Although these preoperative or pretreatment planning devices are not yet part of routine clinical practice, they certainly offer enormous implications for surgical training.

COMPREHENSIVE TRAINING IN TECHNICAL AND NONTECHNICAL SKILLS

Technical and nontechnical skills acquisition is essential for the surgical trainee. With concerns regarding patient safety, new legislation regarding resident work hours, and technological advances allowing for the development of high- and low-fidelity VR simulators, much of the teaching of these skills has moved to the surgical skills laboratory. As Aggarwal described in 2004, the teaching of technical and nontechnical skills should be in a comprehensive, sequential manner.[95] Initially, junior trainees could learn basic surgical skills on a low-fidelity VR simulator. They could then progress to learning the specific steps of an operation on a high-fidelity VR-procedural simulator. Ultimately, they would refine their skills in the simulated operating room, where they would have the opportunity to learn nontechnical skills and practice technical skills under more stressful, realistic conditions. Furthermore, with rapid advancements in technology, it is not inconceivable to imagine surgeons rehearsing operations on an anatomically identical virtual patient before performing the operation in the real world. In addition, although much of the literature focuses on the skill development of the primary surgeon, no surgeon works in isolation, and refocusing training and assessment of teams in addition to individual training is essential to ensure expertise in the operating room. Undre and colleagues[78] describe an initiative to train entire operating room teams in technical and nontechnical skills. In this study, teams were comprised of a surgeon, an anesthetist, an operating-department practitioner, and a scrub nurse. Each team worked through an anesthetic and surgical crisis scenario in the simulated OR. The next conceivable step is taking this type of team training completely to a virtual world. This step would markedly increase the feasibility of team training because of the fact that all parties do not need to be present in the same physical location to participate in the learning experience.

Surgical competence depends on a trainee acquiring technical and nontechnical skills. With the development of virtual-reality simulation, the idea that a trainee should attain a certain level of competence before performing operations on real patients has gained prominence in the literature. The development and maintenance of virtual-reality environments, ranging from a simple VR simulator to a highly complex virtual world, however, is not without cost. It is therefore essential that the validity and the reliability of VR curricula are assessed in the most scientifically rigorous manner. It is time to move beyond the assessment of specific modules of VR simulators, which in the past is where the surgical literature has focused. Indeed, an effective curriculum is far more than simply practice on a simulator. Rather a curriculum is comprised of simulators, specific training schedules, specifically defined levels of expert proficiency, clear assessment parameters, and specific feedback schedules. Examining the effectiveness of these curricula in a holistic manner is necessary to ensure optimal and efficient learning by surgical trainees. Moreover, it is time to investigate further the idea of multidisciplinary team training as an adjunct to the traditional specialty-specific training that currently occurs in most health professional disciplines. Surgery is ultimately a team-based discipline and refining the training in this specialty has the potential to not only increase inter-professional collaboration but also improve patient safety.

REFERENCES

1. Haluck RS, Krummel TM. Computers and virtual reality for surgical education in the 21st century. Arch Surg 2000;135:786.
2. Kneebone R, Nestel D, Wetzel C, et al. The human face of simulation: patient-focused simulation training. Acad Med 2006;81:919.

3. Tavakol M, Mohagheghi MA, Dennick R. Assessing the skills of surgical residents using simulation. J Surg Educ 2008;65:77.
4. Panait L, Bell RL, Roberts KE, et al. Designing and validating a customized virtual reality-based laparoscopic skills curriculum. J Surg Educ 2008;65:413.
5. Schout BM, Hendrikx AJ, Scheele F, et al. Validation and implementation of surgical simulators: a critical review of present, past, and future. Surg Endosc 2010;24(3):536–46.
6. Aggarwal R, Moorthy K, Darzi A. Laparoscopic skills training and assessment. Br J Surg 2004;91:1549.
7. Gallagher AG, Ritter EM, Champion H, et al. Virtual reality simulation for the operating room: proficiency-based training as a paradigm shift in surgical skills training. Ann Surg 2005;241:364.
8. Van Sickle KR, Ritter EM, Smith CD. The pre-trained novice: using simulation-based training to improve learning in the operating room. Surg Innov 2006;13: 198.
9. Gallagher AG, Satava RM. Virtual reality as a metric for the assessment of laparoscopic psychomotor skills. Learning curves and reliability measures. Surg Endosc 2002;16:1746.
10. Gallagher AG, Lederman AB, McGlade K, et al. Discriminative validity of the Minimally Invasive Surgical Trainer in Virtual Reality (MIST-VR) using criteria levels based on expert performance. Surg Endosc 2004;18:660.
11. Grantcharov TP, Funch-Jensen P. Can everyone achieve proficiency with the laparoscopic technique? Learning curve patterns in technical skills acquisition. Am J Surg 2009;197:447.
12. Stefanidis D, Korndorffer JR Jr, Sierra R, et al. Skill retention following proficiency-based laparoscopic simulator training. Surgery 2005;138:165.
13. Gor M, McCloy R, Stone R, et al. Virtual reality laparoscopic simulator for assessment in gynaecology. BJOG 2003;110:181.
14. Sherman V, Feldman LS, Stanbridge D, et al. Assessing the learning curve for the acquisition of laparoscopic skills on a virtual reality simulator. Surg Endosc 2005; 19:678.
15. Aggarwal R, Tully A, Grantcharov T, et al. Virtual reality simulation training can improve technical skills during laparoscopic salpingectomy for ectopic pregnancy. BJOG 2006;113:1382.
16. Buzink SN, Koch AD, Heemskerk J, et al. Acquiring basic endoscopy skills by training on the GI Mentor II. Surg Endosc 2007;21:1996.
17. Colt HG, Crawford SW, Galbraith O 3rd. Virtual reality bronchoscopy simulation: a revolution in procedural training. Chest 2001;120:1333.
18. Eversbusch A, Grantcharov TP. Learning curves and impact of psychomotor training on performance in simulated colonoscopy: a randomized trial using a virtual reality endoscopy trainer. Surg Endosc 2004;18:1514.
19. Jacomides L, Ogan K, Cadeddu JA, et al. Use of a virtual reality simulator for ureteroscopy training. J Urol 2004;171:320.
20. Moorthy K, Smith S, Brown T, et al. Evaluation of virtual reality bronchoscopy as a learning and assessment tool. Respiration 2003;70:195.
21. Wilhelm DM, Ogan K, Roehrborn CG, et al. Assessment of basic endoscopic performance using a virtual reality simulator. J Am Coll Surg 2002;195:675.
22. Ost D, DeRosiers A, Britt EJ, et al. Assessment of a bronchoscopy simulator. Am J Respir Crit Care Med 2001;164:2248.
23. Rowe R, Cohen RA. An evaluation of a virtual reality airway simulator. Anesth Analg 2002;95:62.

24. Park J, MacRae H, Musselman LJ, et al. Randomized controlled trial of virtual reality simulator training: transfer to live patients. Am J Surg 2007;194:205.

25. Ahlberg G, Hultcrantz R, Jaramillo E, et al. Virtual reality colonoscopy simulation: a compulsory practice for the future colonoscopist? Endoscopy 2005;37:1198.

26. Cohen J, Cohen SA, Vora KC, et al. Multicenter, randomized, controlled trial of virtual-reality simulator training in acquisition of competency in colonoscopy. Gastrointest Endosc 2006;64:361.

27. Gerson LB, Van Dam J. A prospective randomized trial comparing a virtual reality simulator to bedside teaching for training in sigmoidoscopy. Endoscopy 2003;35: 569.

28. Di Giulio E, Fregonese D, Casetti T, et al. Training with a computer-based simulator achieves basic manual skills required for upper endoscopy: a randomized controlled trial. Gastrointest Endosc 2004;60:196.

29. Sedlack RE. Validation of computer simulation training for esophagogastroduodenoscopy: pilot study. J Gastroenterol Hepatol 2007;22:1214.

30. Seymour NE, Gallagher AG, Roman SA, et al. Virtual reality training improves operating room performance: results of a randomized, double-blinded study. Ann Surg 2002;236:458.

31. Grantcharov TP, Kristiansen VB, Bendix J, et al. Randomized clinical trial of virtual reality simulation for laparoscopic skills training. Br J Surg 2004;91:146.

32. Carter FJ, Schijven MP, Aggarwal R, et al. Consensus guidelines for validation of virtual reality surgical simulators. Simul Healthc 2006;1:171.

33. Sutherland LM, Middleton PF, Anthony A, et al. Surgical simulation: a systematic review. Ann Surg 2006;243:291.

34. Neequaye SK, Aggarwal R, Van Herzeele I, et al. Endovascular skills training and assessment. J Vasc Surg 2007;46:1055.

35. Datta V, Mandalia M, Mackay S, et al. The Pre-Op flexible sigmoidoscopy trainer. Validation and early evaluation of a virtual reality based system. Surg Endosc 2002;16:1459.

36. Enochsson L, Westman B, Ritter EM, et al. Objective assessment of visuospatial and psychomotor ability and flow of residents and senior endoscopists in simulated gastroscopy. Surg Endosc 2006;20:895.

37. Felsher JJ, Olesevich M, Farres H, et al. Validation of a flexible endoscopy simulator. Am J Surg 2005;189:497.

38. Ferlitsch A, Glauninger P, Gupper A, et al. Evaluation of a virtual endoscopy simulator for training in gastrointestinal endoscopy. Endoscopy 2002;34:698.

39. Koch AD, Buzink SN, Heemskerk J, et al. Expert and construct validity of the Simbionix GI Mentor II endoscopy simulator for colonoscopy. Surg Endosc 2008;22:158.

40. Mahmood T, Darzi A. A study to validate the colonoscopy simulator. Surg Endosc 2003;17:1583.

41. Moorthy K, Munz Y, Jiwanji M, et al. Validity and reliability of a virtual reality upper gastrointestinal simulator and cross validation using structured assessment of individual performance with video playback. Surg Endosc 2004;18:328.

42. Ritter EM, McClusky DA 3rd, Lederman AB, et al. Objective psychomotor skills assessment of experienced and novice flexible endoscopists with a virtual reality simulator. J Gastrointest Surg 2003;7:871.

43. Sedlack RE, Kolars JC. Validation of a computer-based colonoscopy simulator. Gastrointest Endosc 2003;57:214.

44. Dolmans VE, Schout BM, de Beer NA, et al. The virtual reality endourologic simulator is realistic and useful for educational purposes. J Endourol 2009;23:1175.

45. Knudsen BE, Matsumoto ED, Chew BH, et al. A randomized, controlled, prospective study validating the acquisition of percutaneous renal collecting system access skills using a computer based hybrid virtual reality surgical simulator: phase I. J Urol 2006;176:2173.

46. Michel MS, Knoll T, Kohrmann KU, et al. The URO Mentor: development and evaluation of a new computer-based interactive training system for virtual life-like simulation of diagnostic and therapeutic endourological procedures. BJU Int 2002;89:174.

47. Rashid HH, Kowalewski T, Oppenheimer P, et al. The virtual reality transurethral prostatic resection trainer: evaluation of discriminate validity. J Urol 2007;177:2283.

48. Reich O, Noll M, Gratzke C, et al. High-level virtual reality simulator for endourologic procedures of lower urinary tract. Urology 2006;67:1144.

49. Sweet R, Kowalewski T, Oppenheimer P, et al. Face, content and construct validity of the University of Washington virtual reality transurethral prostate resection trainer. J Urol 2004;172:1953.

50. Duffy AJ, Hogle NJ, McCarthy H, et al. Construct validity for the LAPSIM laparoscopic surgical simulator. Surg Endosc 2005;19:401.

51. Eriksen JR, Grantcharov T. Objective assessment of laparoscopic skills using a virtual reality stimulator. Surg Endosc 2005;19:1216.

52. Gallagher AG, Richie K, McClure N, et al. Objective psychomotor skills assessment of experienced, junior, and novice laparoscopists with virtual reality. World J Surg 2001;25:1478.

53. Grantcharov TP, Bardram L, Funch-Jensen P, et al. Learning curves and impact of previous operative experience on performance on a virtual reality simulator to test laparoscopic surgical skills. Am J Surg 2003;185:146.

54. McDougall EM, Corica FA, Boker JR, et al. Construct validity testing of a laparoscopic surgical simulator. J Am Coll Surg 2006;202:779.

55. Schreuder HW, van Dongen KW, Roeleveld SJ, et al. Face and construct validity of virtual reality simulation of laparoscopic gynecologic surgery. Am J Obstet Gynecol 2009;200:540.e1.

56. van Dongen KW, Tournoij E, van der Zee DC, et al. Construct validity of the LapSim: can the LapSim virtual reality simulator distinguish between novices and experts? Surg Endosc 2007;21:1413.

57. Woodrum DT, Andreatta PB, Yellamanchilli RK, et al. Construct validity of the LapSim laparoscopic surgical simulator. Am J Surg 2006;191:28.

58. Kundhal PS, Grantcharov TP. Psychomotor performance measured in a virtual environment correlates with technical skills in the operating room. Surg Endosc 2009;23:645.

59. Moorthy K, Munz Y, Orchard TR, et al. An innovative method for the assessment of skills in lower gastrointestinal endoscopy. Surg Endosc 2004;18:1613.

60. Seymour NE. VR to OR: a review of the evidence that virtual reality simulation improves operating room performance. World J Surg 2008;32:182.

61. Gardner R, Raemer DB. Simulation in obstetrics and gynecology. Obstet Gynecol Clin North Am 2008;35:97.

62. Munz Y, Almoudaris AM, Moorthy K, et al. Curriculum-based solo virtual reality training for laparoscopic intracorporeal knot tying: objective assessment of the transfer of skill from virtual reality to reality. Am J Surg 2007;193:774.

63. Ericsson KA. Deliberate practice and the acquisition and maintenance of expert performance in medicine and related domains. Acad Med 2004;79:S70.

64. Moulton CA, Dubrowski A, Macrae H, et al. Teaching surgical skills: what kind of practice makes perfect?: a randomized, controlled trial. Ann Surg 2006;244:400.

65. Mackay S, Morgan P, Datta V, et al. Practice distribution in procedural skills training: a randomized controlled trial. Surg Endosc 2002;16:957.
66. Ali MR, Mowery Y, Kaplan B, et al. Training the novice in laparoscopy. More challenge is better. Surg Endosc 2002;16:1732.
67. Stefanidis D, Heniford BT. The formula for a successful laparoscopic skills curriculum. Arch Surg 2009;144:77.
68. Kruglikova I, Grantcharov TP, Drewes AM, et al. Assessment of early learning curves among nurses and physicians using a high-fidelity virtual-reality colonoscopy simulator. Surg Endosc 2010;24(2):366–70.
69. Porte MC, Xeroulis G, Reznick RK, et al. Verbal feedback from an expert is more effective than self-accessed feedback about motion efficiency in learning new surgical skills. Am J Surg 2007;193:105.
70. Xeroulis GJ, Park J, Moulton CA, et al. Teaching suturing and knot-tying skills to medical students: a randomized controlled study comparing computer-based video instruction and (concurrent and summary) expert feedback. Surgery 2007;141:442.
71. Christian CK, Gustafson ML, Roth EM, et al. A prospective study of patient safety in the operating room. Surgery 2006;139:159.
72. Mishra A, Catchpole K, Dale T, et al. The influence of non-technical performance on technical outcome in laparoscopic cholecystectomy. Surg Endosc 2008; 22:68.
73. Stevenson KS, Gibson SC, MacDonald D, et al. Measurement of process as quality control in the management of acute surgical emergencies. Br J Surg 2007;94:376.
74. Yule S, Flin R, Paterson-Brown S, et al. Non-technical skills for surgeons in the operating room: a review of the literature. Surgery 2006;139:140.
75. Moorthy K, Munz Y, Adams S, et al. A human factors analysis of technical and team skills among surgical trainees during procedural simulations in a simulated operating theatre. Ann Surg 2005;242:631.
76. Moorthy K, Munz Y, Forrest D, et al. Surgical crisis management skills training and assessment: a simulation [corrected]-based approach to enhancing operating room performance. Ann Surg 2006;244:139.
77. Powers KA, Rehrig ST, Irias N, et al. Simulated laparoscopic operating room crisis: an approach to enhance the surgical team performance. Surg Endosc 2008;22:885.
78. Undre S, Koutantji M, Sevdalis N, et al. Multidisciplinary crisis simulations: the way forward for training surgical teams. World J Surg 2007;31:1843.
79. Paige J, Kozmenko V, Morgan B, et al. From the flight deck to the operating room: an initial pilot study of the feasibility and potential impact of true interdisciplinary team training using high-fidelity simulation. J Surg Educ 2007;64:369.
80. Karim Qayumi A, Qayumi T. Computer-assisted learning: CyberPatient–a step in the future of surgical education. J Invest Surg 1999;12:307.
81. Mayrose J, Myers JW. Endotracheal intubation: application of virtual reality to emergency medical services education. Simul Healthc 2007;2:231.
82. Schwid HA, Rooke GA, Michalowski P, et al. Screen-based anesthesia simulation with debriefing improves performance in a mannequin-based anesthesia simulator. Teach Learn Med 2001;13:92.
83. Vash JH, Yunesian M, Shariati M, et al. Virtual patients in undergraduate surgery education: a randomized controlled study. ANZ J Surg 2007;77:54.
84. Youngblood P, Heinrichs L, Cornelius C, et al. Designing case-based learning for virtual worlds. Simul Healthc 2007;2:246.

85. LeRoy Heinrichs W, Youngblood P, Harter PM, et al. Simulation for team training and assessment: case studies of online training with virtual worlds. World J Surg 2008;32:161.

86. Boulos MN, Hetherington L, Wheeler S. Second Life: an overview of the potential of 3-D virtual worlds in medical and health education. Health Info Libr J 2007; 24:233.

87. Hansen MM. Versatile, immersive, creative and dynamic virtual 3-D healthcare learning environments: a review of the literature. J Med Internet Res 2008; 10:e26.

88. Cohen ZA, Henry JH, McCarthy DM, et al. Computer simulations of patellofemoral joint surgery. Patient-specific models for tuberosity transfer. Am J Sports Med 2003;31:87.

89. Luboz V, Chabanas M, Swider P, et al. Orbital and maxillofacial computer aided surgery: patient-specific finite element models to predict surgical outcomes. Comput Methods Biomech Biomed Engin 2005;8:259.

90. Ng I, Hwang PY, Kumar D, et al. Surgical planning for microsurgical excision of cerebral arterio-venous malformations using virtual reality technology. Acta Neurochir (Wien) 2009;151:453.

91. Roguin A, Beyar R. Real case virtual reality training prior to carotid artery stenting. Catheter Cardiovasc Interv 2010;75(2):279–82.

92. Soler L, Marescaux J. Patient-specific surgical simulation. World J Surg 2008;32: 208.

93. Sierra R, Dimaio SP, Wada J, et al. Patient specific simulation and navigation of ventriculoscopic interventions. Stud Health Technol Inform 2007;125:433.

94. Sadiq SK, Mazzeo MD, Zasada SJ, et al. Patient-specific simulation as a basis for clinical decision-making. Philos Transact A Math Phys Eng Sci 2008;366:3199.

95. Aggarwal R, Undre S, Moorthy K, et al. The simulated operating theatre: comprehensive training for surgical teams. Qual Saf Health care 2004;13(Suppl 1):i27.

The Role of Simulation in Certification

Jo Buyske, MD

KEYWORDS

- American Board of Surgery • ABS • Certification
- Simulation • Surgical simulation

The American Board of Surgery (ABS) is a private, nonprofit organization that was chartered in 1937. It is part of a larger umbrella group of medical boards called the American Board of Medical Specialties. The original charter of the ABS states that it exists to protect the public and improve the specialty. The ABS Booklet of Information, published annually, further notes that the specific objective of the ABS is "to pass judgment on the education, training, and knowledge of broadly qualified and responsible surgeons." This is done by conducting examinations, issuing certificates to candidates meeting the board's requirements, and working to improve and broaden opportunities for the graduate education and training of surgeons. Until recently, this process did not include using simulation as part of the education or assessment of surgeons.

Simulation and assessment of surgeons would seem to be a perfect match, and there is much enthusiasm around the concept. We all know that the airline industry uses simulation in training and testing pilots. It follows that other fields that combine knowledge, experience, and technical skill should also be taught and tested in simulators. It may come to pass that we will use simulators to formally test the various components of surgery in the future, but we are not there yet.

The fields of surgical simulation and virtual reality have developed in silos around teaching and training. At every large surgical meeting, there will be exhibitors and lecturers demonstrating their particular virtual reality program or simulation model. Often these models are well thought out and developed. More than a few teaching programs use either homegrown or purchased simulation models in some aspect of resident training. Few of these models have attained widespread use in heterogenous settings. This is a significant issue, in that the limited penetration of any given model has prevented true assessment of the outcome of training on those models. In training, it may be enough to pass a test of reason; if the teachers feel that the students are doing better using a given simulation model, that is good enough. For high-stakes

No funding support was received for this document.
American Board of Surgery, University of Pennsylvania School of Medicine, 1617 John F. Kennedy Boulevard, Suite 860, Philadelphia, PA 19103, USA
E-mail address: jbuyske@absurgery.org

assessment such as that involved in the ABS certification process, however, standardization and validation are essential.

The ABS assessments rest on completion of an Accreditation Council for Graduate Medical Education (ACGME)–accredited residency program in the United States or Canada, testimonial from the program director of that program, a case list showing adequate volume and breadth, and 2 tests: the Qualifying Examination, which is a computer-based multiple-choice test that focuses on testing knowledge, and the Certifying Examination (CE), which is an oral examination that focuses on the integration of that knowledge to make decisions. Neither examination uses virtual reality. The CE might loosely be described as a simulation, in that patient scenarios are verbally presented to the examinee, who then develops a plan for diagnosis and management, asking for and incorporating new information and changes in the scenario as it unfolds. There is, however, no mannequin or computer involved and no attempt to pretend that the case is live.

In June 2008, the ABS board of directors voted to include simulation in the requirements for certification for the first time. Successful completion of the Fundamentals of Laparoscopic Surgery (FLS) (Society of Gastrointestinal and Endoscopic Surgeons and American College of Surgeons) as well as Advanced Trauma Life Support (American College of Surgeons) and Advanced Cardiovascular Life Support (American Heart Association) became the requirement for certification for those surgical residents finishing in 2010 or later. These programs are not administered as part of an ABS examination, but rather through the societies that developed them, and a certificate of successful completion of the program is then presented to the ABS as part of the application portfolio.

FLS uses simulation to teach and assess basic skills in laparoscopic surgery. The metrics for teaching and assessment have been vetted internationally. The test-taking platform is standardized, affordable, mass produced, and portable. The standards for testing have been distilled down to a program that allows nonsurgeon proctors to grade an examinee's performance. An ongoing program to train proctors has allowed the examination to be given at convenient locations and times all across the country.

For simulation to assume a formal role in the assessment of surgeons, models need to be developed that meet a similar description. The area being assessed must fall in the broad domain of surgery and must be essential and common enough to justify the testing requirement. There must be expert agreement as to the importance of the subject matter. The test must be validated in multiple settings by multiple users and during a period of time. The test equipment must be accessible to the entire population of surgeons who seek board certification, either because it is portable and affordable or because it is distributed strategically throughout the country and made available. The test metrics must show interrater reliability, such that proctors throughout the country can confidently give a reliable score to examinees. Last, ideally the test should be one that can be administered as a prerequisite to taking the ABS examinations, not as part of the examinations themselves.

The General Surgery Milestones Project is a joint project between the ACGME and the ABS. The purpose of the project is to identify milestones along the road of surgical training and to quantify what residents are learning and how they are progressing. Milestones might include knowledge tests, skill tests, clinical observations, or other accomplishments. One can see a role for simulation as a milestone. For example, it might be reasonable that to assess a resident's training in surgical critical care, in addition to being exposed to a certain number and variety of cases and the time-based training of a 2- or 3-month rotation, the resident might be required to pass a simulation involving a postoperative patient who has cardiac ischemia. Mannequins and computer-driven simulation might be used to provide a standardized scenario in which a resident could be assessed in multiple arenas. Medical knowledge, judgment, team-based action, leadership, flexibility, communication, and professionalism might all be quantified in such a setting. Documentation of successful completion of such a scenario could be a required component of residency. Residents wishing to transfer from 1 program to another would have to show a portfolio of completed milestones to document their proper training level. At the completion of training, the entire completed portfolio would be required as part of the application for the qualifying examination in surgery. Thus, simulation becomes not part of the examination process but rather an integrated part of the ongoing assessment of surgeons that culminates in board examinations.

The technology exists to make exciting changes in assessment of the myriad skills that go into being a fully trained surgeon. The challenge lies in the details of sorting through the richness of opportunity out there and validating a few models and measurements that can fairly be applied as a yardstick against which all can be measured.

Emerging Trends that Herald the Future of Surgical Simulation

Richard M. Satava, MD[a,b,*]

KEYWORDS

- Surgical simulation • Simulation science
- Surgical education • Skills curricula

There is now an acceptance, based on validated curricula and simulators,[1] that patient safety is improved through simulation-based training. This acceptance is based on the recent adoption of a myriad of simulation technologies and a revolution in surgical education. The last such revolution was 100 years ago with the Flexner report[2] in 1910, which was driven by a need to change the apprenticeship model toward a more consistent and comprehensive training model through the establishment of more formal residency training programs. Although significant, this change continued the emphasis on training the surgeon rather than on patient safety.

This situation has evolved into the current process of training and evaluation of surgeons, based on subjective judgment (and a few objective measures such question and answer, case-based discourse, tests, and so forth), which focused on knowledge. Skills-based training and assessment has previously been accomplished exclusively by subjective appraisal in the hospital or operating room (OR), or based on the number of surgical procedures (without any measures of performance).

We are in the midst of a new revolution in surgical education, which is being "opportunity driven" by external forces—principally by the introduction of new technologies and the political desire to ensure patient safety. The political forces have been caused by a more informed public (patients) as well as health care activism. These issues are critical in the acceptance of changes, but are not addressed herein. The technologies,

The opinions or assertions contained herein are the private views of the author and are not to be construed as official, or as reflecting the views of the Departments of the Army, Navy or Air Force, the Defense Advanced Research Projects Agency, or the Department of Defense.

This is a declared work of the US Government and as such is not subject to copyright protection in the United States.

[a] Department of Surgery, University of Washington Medical Center, 1959 Pacific Street NE, Seattle, WA 98195, USA
[b] US Army Medical Research and Material Command, Ft Detrick, MD, USA
* Department of Surgery, University of Washington Medical Center, 1959 Pacific Street NE, Seattle, WA 98195.
E-mail address: rsatava@u.washington.edu

Surg Clin N Am 90 (2010) 623–633
doi:10.1016/j.suc.2010.02.002
0039-6109/10/$ – see front matter. Published by Elsevier Inc.

surgical.theclinics.com

principally in simulation (broadly defined) include not only "simulators" but also the curricula with assessment tools. It is the convergence of these 2 aspects, the introduction of simulation for skills training and the structured objective assessment of skills performance (including cognitive skills such as communication) with benchmark metrics that has enabled simulation to transform surgical education from subjective judgment to objective measurement of performance.

The traditional psychomotor skills simulation technology has been based on physical models and animal parts (pig trotters, rendered intestines, and so forth), whereas the emerging simulation employs manikins, recent computer-based interactive programs, and a variety of virtual reality (VR) simulations, with variations such as full head-mounted displays, augmented reality, and hybrid VR with physical models. The new curricula have been focused on basic skills, a few advanced skills, and team training. Within the past decade, patient actors have begun to be used to teach elements of history and physical examination, as well as assessment of communication skills and professionalism in what is termed the Objective Structured Clinical Exam (OSCE). In 1997, Resnick and colleagues[3] developed a formalized curriculum methodology to quantitatively assess performance of psychomotor skills, entitled the Objective Structured Assessment of Technical Skills (OSATS). The following year, Derossis and colleagues[4] adapted the methodology to a specific curriculum for laparoscopic surgery, called the Fundamentals of Laparoscopic Surgery (FLS). Together, the OSCE and OSATS have turned the subjective training and evaluation of psychomotor, cognitive, and communication skills into a method of quantifying performance with measurable results. Even more important is that by measuring the performance of experienced and expert surgeons with these methods, benchmarks of competent performance could be established. Such progress has led to the profound revolution of "training to proficiency" (or competency), meaning that residents are no longer trained for a specified time (ie, a few days) before performing a procedure on patients. Instead the residents are trained for whatever length of time is required to reach the benchmark measures, with some residents finishing faster and others taking longer; however, no resident is permitted to perform a procedure on a patient until the criterion benchmark is reached. This change in education, while not guaranteeing patient safety, clearly improves it, as has been demonstrated in numerous studies on the reduction of errors and improvement in the efficiency after training on a simulator. This fact should come as no surprise, because most other professions (such as aviation, military, and so forth) have been using these methods for decades.

MANDATES

As indicated above, it has taken more than 15 years since the beginning of the first surgical simulators[5] to acquire enough evidence to prove the effectiveness of training using simulators with objective assessment to proficiency.[1] The result has been that the surgical education and certifying community has issued mandates that require the implementation of surgical simulation into residency training. The first such mandate came in 2003 from the Accreditation Council on Graduate Medical Education (ACGME), in conjunction with the American Board of Medical Specialties (ABMS), by redefining in precise terms the 6 competencies that must be taught, measured, and certified: Knowledge, patient care, communication and interpersonal skills, professionalism, systems-based practice, and lifelong learning. It is noted that only the first 2 competencies had traditionally been formally taught. The remainder had either been informally taught during rounds or in the OR, or had not even been acknowledged as important aspects of surgical education.

In 2008, the second mandate was issued by the surgical Residency Review Committee (RRC) of the ACGME.[6] This mandate requires that all surgical residency programs must have access to "… simulation and skills laboratories." The implications of this mandate are profound, once again emphasizing the importance of quantifiable skills training in the safe environment of a laboratory setting: it is no longer acceptable to "practice on" a patient; rather, skills competency must first be learned through simulation.

In 2009, the third mandate was issued by the American Board of Surgery (ABS).[7] Convinced of the significant improvement in training and in safety as demonstrated by analogy to other industries that use simulation, and by the unequivocal validation of FLS, the ABS now requires that applicants for "… the General Surgery Qualifying Examination must … provide documentation of successful completion [of FLS] with their application." Otherwise the application will be considered incomplete and returned to the candidate, who will not be permitted to sit for the examination to receive ABS Certification.

In addition, ever since 1979 the ABS has limited the certification to a 10-year period, and thus all Board Certified Surgeons must be recertified every 10 years—an acknowledgment of how perishable medical knowledge is and how rapidly technology is changing the practice of surgery. The process associated with this requirement is referred to as Maintenance of Certification (MOC). Over the intervening years, most other specialties have instituted their own policies for MOC. More important is that recently, the various other certifying boards of the ABMS have not only issued their own mandates for MOC but are actually shortening the period for recertification, such as the requirements of the American Board of Pediatrics (ABP) for "…5-year MOC cycle [which] begins January 1, 2010." On the ABP Web site, pediatricians will be listed as ABP certified and designated as "Meeting current requirements for maintenance of certification… for a length of 5 years."[8] It is highly likely that the ABS will be soon requiring the MOC at the 5 year period, and will be including skills training beyond the initial FLS.

SIMULATION CENTERS

In response to these new mandates regarding simulation centers, specific skills courses, and the need for MOC, the American College of Surgeons (ACS) has responded in a twofold manner, aiming for: (1) development of a certification process to guarantee the quality of the training in a simulation center and (2) development of a standardized skills curriculum that can meet the requirements of the RRC and ABS.

The certification of a surgical simulation center is voluntary, though clearly such a certificate would be advantageous when the routine RRC review of a surgical training program is performed. The ACS has established a stringent application and survey process (similar to the evaluation conducted by the RRC, which includes a 1-day on-site survey by 2 surveyors) that can result in a certificate as an Accredited Educational Institute (AEI). The ACS has purposefully designed the requirements to include training of multiple professionals (physicians, nurses, pharmacists, and so forth) to not only emphasize the importance of "interprofessional" training as a critical component of performance as a team (see later discussion) but also to include documentation of training to proficiency with longitudinal (annual) analysis of the quality of the training provided. The process also includes specific resource requirements (such as minimal amount of space, number of personnel, types of simulation equipment, types of curricula, and so forth). As of the end of 2009 there are 48 AEI, which include 8 centers outside the United States. These institutions formed the Consortium of

ACS-AEI, which held the first annual Consortium meeting in September 2008. The strategy of this consortium is to develop a more uniform approach to surgical (skills) education in 3 specific areas:

1. *Development of a single Web-based Learning Management System (LMS).* Such a database will include all the training documentation of each resident in each training program to establish a national norm of training against which each consortium member can measure their performance. In addition, the database will include all the different courses (and curricula) taught by all of the consortium simulation centers. Analyses of the LMS database will permit the Consortium to determine where there are curriculum "gaps" that need to be addressed. All data that are maintained in the consortium database will be de-identified for anonymity to ensure compliance with the Healthcare Information Privacy and Portability Act (HIPPA).
2. *Coordination of the development of curricula.* To date, there has been no coordination of available curricula, and the result is that many different curricula (with different outcomes measures) exist for the same procedures, such as laparoscopic cholecystectomy and airway intubation. In addition, there is no uniform method for developing a curriculum. There are many areas where curricula need to be developed, and it would be of great advantage for a number of the members to collaborate on developing a single specific curriculum that is then adopted by the remaining members of the Consortium, thus leading to a more standardized overall surgical curriculum on a national (or international) level. Why a resident trained at one institution should have a completely different education and different assessment criteria than another resident at a different institution for exactly the same surgical procedures is incomprehensible. Even considering the different available teaching styles, individual patient variation, and surgeon preferences, there should be at least a common "generic" approach to a surgical procedure, which then can be amplified (once the standard approach is learned) to the faculty members' preferred approach. Imagine what would occur if every pilot would have their own way of navigating a commercial jet without air route regulation and air traffic control rules; specific flight paths must be followed to maintain safety, even though pilots fly their aircraft slightly different from one another. An added benefit of joint development of curriculum is that a multi-institutional validation study (with enough subjects to provide statistical significance) can be performed in a much quicker time frame.
3. *Collaboration in research.* In much the same manner by which validation studies can be coordinated, a research agenda is being developed for new areas of simulation, including not only innovative simulators but also new types of curricula, assessment processes, and even training programs. Such an agenda will identify the areas where research needs to be performed, and help coordinate collaborative studies. Such multi-institutional studies, under the imprimatur of the ACS-AEI, would have a significant competitive advantage when applying for federal funding.

The second response by the ACS to the mandates is to work within the surgical education community and to develop in collaboration with the ABS and the Association of Program Directors in Surgery (APDS) an initial set of curricula: Basic Skills, Advanced Procedures, and Team Training. These curricula can become the foundation of the training programs of the Consortium of ACS-AEI, and may well become the basis for skills training that will be required by the ABS for Board Certification.

The ACGME, RRC, ACS, APDS, ABS, and the entire surgical education community has embarked on a strategic revamping of the educational process for residents and surgeons, including not only initial training, but "retraining," such as MOC for established surgeons. The same curriculum that is being developed for MOC can also be used (perhaps with minor modifications) for the retraining of established surgeons when returning from a prolonged absence (see later discussion). More important than improving the quality and efficiency of training, implicit in this endeavor is that patient safety can be improved through a more scientific approach to surgical skills training. It is also envisioned that some of the constraints to surgical education that result from the imposition of limitations to the work hours of residents can be relieved through more efficient training in a simulation environment. This strategy is especially applicable to the basic skills and team training, where the "learning curve" can be moved from the bedside to the laboratory, thereby decreasing likelihood of patient error in the clinical setting.

A final trend that is occurring because of the establishment of skills training centers is that the courses and training programs that have been instituted for surgical residents are being "moved down" to the medical student level. The anticipated consequence is that when a medical student enters residency training, the basic skills will already have been learned including inculcating team training and a "culture of safety," and more advanced training can begin earlier in their program. With this exposure, a self-selection effect could affect the make-up of the applicant pool to residency. In addition, as part of the application to surgical residency, an objective evaluation of prospective residents' skills (in addition to their knowledge base) will be available.

STATE OF THE ART

To understand where the future of surgical simulation may be heading, the current state of the art needs to be reviewed, thereby providing a baseline against which the emerging technologies can be compared in terms of their likelihood of success as well as the timing of their adoption. This comparison provides a pragmatic approach to monitoring and implementing the new mandates, technologies, and processes.

Mandates

The current mandates and policies (see earlier discussion) are limited to the Surgical RRC of the ACGME and the ACS/ABS. Other surgical specialties have not produced such requirements, although almost all specialties (both medical and surgical) are addressing the issue. The MOC mandate currently stands at recertification every 10 years and there are no policies regarding other aspects of retraining. Granting of hospital privileges remains at the local hospital level, and there are no standardized requirements for documentation of skills training, currency in procedures performed, and evidence of certified training in a new procedure.

Technologies

The areas and technologies where simulation is being used are for basic skills (the 20 core skills identified by the ACS/APDS/ABS), a few advanced procedures, and team training. Most simulators and skills curricula are for general surgery, anesthesiology, and nursing, although there are some simulators in flexible endoscopy, urology, and obstetrics/gynecology. The greatest amount of skills training is being conducted at the basic skills level, using simple, cost-effective physical models. However, almost all laparoscopic surgery training is being conducted with videoscopic trainer models, VR simulators, or animal models. There are very sophisticated VR simulators for endovascular procedures, which even include patient-specific simulations. Manikin simulators have been used for specific technical skills (airway management, induction of anesthesia, conscious sedation), but their most frequent use is for clinical management and team training. The training and assessment of the nontechnical skills of the 6 ACGME competencies (physical examination, communication, and so forth) is mainly through the use of OSCE with patient actors, though some is being conducted with manikins. Assessment tools include OSATS, OSCE, and FLS. Others are under development.

Research

As indicated earlier, research is not coordinated, is driven by individuals who are inspired to create a simulation (or simulator), and frequently duplicates or competes with other existing simulators. There had previously been a flurry of activity in developing surgical simulators. However, due to recent reductions in available funding, that activity has slowed appreciably. The new mandates have provided an incentive for training programs to ensure adequate resources as well as simulators.

Clinical Practice

At present, the only routine application of simulation to clinical practice is in vascular procedures or in complex liver operations. Professor Marescaux of the IRCAD institute in Strasbourg, France has used simulation to preplan and rehearse clinical liver resection for hepatic cancer.[9]

Because the 6 ACGME competencies are so critical, the following are examples of the types of simulation used to specifically address the different competencies:

1. *Knowledge*. This is principally traditional teaching through didactic lectures, rounds, and instruction during surgery. Web-based, interactive curricula improve the quality of the training by including multimedia, especially video and animated graphics, in the didactic portions.
2. *Patient care*. Although traditional rounds, operating on patients, and OSCE still comprise the most common method of training, patient care is where most of the tasks and specific skills are conducted on manikins, models, and VR simulators. Manikins are used for teaching airway management/anesthesia skills and team training; physical models are principally used for basic technical skills and specific tasks (such as chest tube); and mechanical or VR simulators are used for specific tasks and simple procedures (such as laparoscopic cholecystectomy). Training for open surgery and advanced procedures is still performed on animal models because the simulators are not yet of sufficiently high fidelity to provide the necessary level of realism.
3. *Communication and interpersonal skills*. Today, these skills require observation and grading (with objective check lists and global rating scores). The skills can be trained and assessed using the OSCE format or manikins. There is a growing number of curricula to incorporate simulation of these skills, but even "objective assessment" includes the subjective placement of an observed action into a Likert (or similar) scale to attempt to quantify the performance.
4. *Professionalism*. This is a very difficult skill to teach, and is traditionally acquired by mentorship and direct observation of effective leadership, as well as moral and ethical behavior in a faculty member. Some aspects of professionalism can be taught didactically, while others can be elicited in an OSCE type of activity.
5. *Systems-based practice*. This new requirement can be taught through manikin-based team training. There needs to be a clearer definition of what is meant by

systems-based learning that is accepted across specialties and, if possible, metrics developed so that a curriculum can be designed.
6. *Practice-based learning and improvement.* Other than attempting to adapt OSCE to continuing improvement, there are no curricula that address this issue. This is principally an issue of documentation of training and practice outcomes (eg, morbidity and mortality conference, quality assurance assessment), with evidence that surgeons have changed/improved their practice outcomes based on reflection of their practice.

It is clear from these examples of the use of simulation that not all of the required skills will be solely achieved by the use of simulation, though it is likely that some new creative approaches will emerge.

FUTURE DIRECTIONS
Mandates

There can be little doubt that in the near and distant future, the number of mandates will grow in response to the public's insatiable desire for transparency and the profession's agreement for accountability to ensure patient safety. The specialty societies will eventually all adopt some of the simulation technologies to augment both training and assessment—these will first be required by the training programs, and then by the representative boards for certification. MOC will move to shorter time spans, very likely every 5 years, with the possibility of every 3 years or even being automatically generated in "real time" during both practice and laboratory training. In addition to the specialty societies and certification boards, the local hospital privileging and credentialing committees will be adopting more comprehensive documentation of training, which will apply not only to initial and renewal privileging but also to MOC and retraining. Eventually every category of procedure that is requested will require presentation of a certificate documenting competency. Likewise, procedures that are not performed frequently (eg, failure to perform to a desired number per year) will require either remediation or retraining. As more requirements are added, increasingly sophisticated simulation methods will become a very attractive alternative to practice on patients.

Very similar to MOC, the retraining will be applied to many special circumstances, such as when returning from absences due to sabbatical, maternity/paternity leave, administrative and nonmedical education degrees, and duty to country. The latter is currently a significant issue for both the military and the civilian reserve physicians who are deployed to support combat operations. These surgeons are torn from the daily practice and usually begin treating patients with very different diseases or injuries from their specialty practice. The military experience indicates that it takes from 3 to 6 months for a returning surgeon to "reintegrate" back to their peacetime practice.

Technologies

In response to continued pressure to completely avoid the use of humans and animals for training, use of simulation will continue to increase. The most basic change will be the development of "virtual cadavers" based on 3-dimensional reconstructed tomographic images of a specific cadaver. This virtual cadaver can be shared among a group of students who can repeatedly practice "virtual dissection" before dissecting an actual cadaver. Over time a huge library of scans of hundreds of variations of critical anatomy will be acquired, and it may be possible to stop nearly all cadaver use at this level of medical education. With such a large library of virtual anatomy, students can learn about (and virtually dissect) all the different variations, anomalies, and diseases of every organ system. Thus a very structured curriculum can be created to ensure that each student learns about all the major variations, not just the singular characteristics of the cadaver to which they happen to be assigned. This same library can be used for residents to practice virtual operations, to gain expertise by performing the same operations with many variations, and thus complete operations without making errors (proficiency). This practice will facilitate a surgeon's progression from competency to mastery through "experience" and exposure to a large number of variations of the basic procedure. Patient-specific computed tomography scans (with consent) could expand the library as well as increase the number of variations that would be available for training complex procedures for both residents and practicing surgeons. By the time such a library is collected, simulation technology will accrue sufficient increases in fidelity to make even complex procedures possible.

In a similar fashion, patient actors in the OSCE will be mainly replaced by "virtual patients," which will have not only clinically relevant ("intelligent") responses to questions in the history and the ability to provide physical examination sensory input, but also will include appropriate human social, behavioral, and cultural (HSBC) responses with realistic emotional representation in speech, facial expression, pose, and nonverbal cues. The current research in HSBC in training military and civilian personnel deployed overseas is making extraordinary progress in creating "virtual actors" that behave and respond in a lifelike manner nearly indistinguishable from an actual person. During surveys for the ACS-AEI, the author has queried numerous institutions as to the cost of employing patient actors for OSCE, as well as the use of cadavers for medical student and procedure training. Of note, the range for both of the types of training/assessment is from $200,000 to $800,000 per year, depending on the amount of such training that the specific center performs. It is clear that dramatic decreases in overall center expense can be achieved by replacing most (not all) of such training with virtual cadavers or virtual patients. In addition, education will be enhanced by the development of huge libraries of numerous variations, able to provide the substrate for a well-structured curriculum that will include all the important facets of a disease state, and not continue the current hit-or-miss approach whereby the student only gets to learn (and be assessed) by the cadaver, actor, or on-service patient who happens to be available at the time.

VR simulators have also been adapted for preoperative warm-up immediately before a procedure. Kahol and colleagues[10] have demonstrated in the laboratory a decrease in operating time and errors by warming up for 15 minutes before performing a procedure. This is an example of a priori knowledge that has been implemented in many other professions (symphony, baseball, basketball, dance, and so forth), and demonstrates how warming up before a demanding activity can dramatically enhance performance. This improvement effect persists for about 30 minutes, and enhances performance of novices and experts alike. In addition, preoperative warm-up is needed before every procedure because the increased psychomotor performance and increased attention and near-term memory do not carry over from one operation to the next, mainly due to the waning of the improvement effect beyond 30 minutes.

Manikins will all become tetherless and reach greater degrees of visual and physical (eg, tissue characteristics, bleeding) fidelity to a point where they will incorporate not only physiology feedback, but enable performance of more advanced procedures as well. Team training is moving out from the laboratory and into the hospital environment (in situ training) by placing the manikin in an intensive care unit (ICU) bed, in the emergency room (ER), or in other actual environments. Preliminary investigations demonstrate that in situ training is valuable in identifying system errors, in addition to enhancing communication and professionalism. Because the simulation center has all the equipment, drugs, and instruments correctly prepared for the training episode, system errors such as the wrong dose of medication stored at the nursing station, or not having the correct connector or instrument available on the floor are not discovered during laboratory training, but rapidly appear during in situ training. In addition, interprofessional team training will be extended to train and assess continuity of care. The current curricula for team training in the ER, ICU, and OR situation will be strung together to ensure the proper "hand-off" of the patient from one team to the next. A typical type of scenario could include stabilization of the patient by the ER team, hand-off to the OR team, then safe transfer of the patient to the ICU postoperatively. Key issues include connectivity of instrumentation (eg, ensure the endotracheal tube can connect to the ventilator), transmission of critical information (laboratory data, previously administered drugs, and so forth), and communication of completed or continued treatment protocols.

Tele-simulation is being explored to provide at a remote location the same level of training that occurs at a major medical center location. With a smaller staff, a remote hospital coordinates with the director and faculty of the simulation center to conduct a training course at the local institution over the Internet. Depending on the type of course, a simulator or manikin can be shipped to the remote location (reducing procurement costs associated with very expensive equipment intended for only occasional use). Once the remote staff is trained, the large expense in time, travel, and actual cost for repeated training and MOC can be substantially decreased by having them participate in teaching roles in training and evaluation of additional students/faculty at the remote location. Tele-simulation is clearly going to be a major issue as the need for MOC compliance significantly increases.

Crossing the boundaries between virtual patients/cadavers and tele-simulation and training, there will be an increase in the use of virtual environments (VE), such as Second Life (SL). This technology can provide a complete representation of a simulation center or conference room on the Internet in one of the VEs that are now commercially available, the best known of which is the free SL "world." Different from games that are played on the Internet, SL only provides the "world" or terrain and the "tools" such as virtual person (avatar), methods of "travel" throughout the world, and methods of interaction with various objects such as simulators, projections of powerpoint presentations, and video clips. Individuals can build their specific place, such as a store to actually purchase "clothes" to change the appearance of one's avatar, or a conference room to hold virtual meetings, and in particular complete buildings that can exactly replicate an actual simulation center. Then the students can come to the virtual center and practice the simulation without leaving home or the office. While this is available at a relatively simplistic level at this time, rapid technological advances are increasing the fidelity (and believability) of such VEs. Although most training will not occur in a virtual simulation center, the new generation of residents and surgeons are embracing this technology and are very comfortable working there. At present the military has a program called Virtually Home for soldiers with traumatic brain injury and posttraumatic stress disorder (TBI/PTSD) in which the warriors are able to return to their home city and visit daily the virtual "warrior transition unit" office to participate in their military duties, or have a rehabilitation session with their doctor, psychologist, or rehabilitation therapist.

Research

The most important aspects of research will be identifying the "gaps" in the current training and assessment capabilities and products, and then to establish a coordinated, multi-institutional approach that will provide more researchers to solve the problems as well as a larger pool of subjects to validate the efficacy. Such an approach also will (hopefully) reduce the redundant efforts of many different researchers and companies that are developing curricula/simulators. The current model has resulted in different outcomes measures and assessment tools, and dramatically different training for the same procedures at many different institutions. This situation can be improved with establishment of a more uniform training curriculum. It is essential to reach consensus on core curriculum issues that can provide a common foundation for all surgeons, and then for individual institutions/faculty to modify such a foundation to local needs or preferences.

Clinical Practice

While the value of simulation-based training and assessment in the laboratory environment will continue to provide an enormous benefit for quality of health care and patient safety, the greater long-term benefit will be realized as simulation becomes integrated into clinical practice. The procedures practiced in the laboratory will soon be instantiated in clinical practice as patient-specific preoperative planning and surgical rehearsal. Eventually, nearly every procedure will be rehearsed on the image of the patient just before the surgeon conducts the actual procedure on the patient. Following the rehearsal, preoperative warm-up will be used to adequately prime the surgeon for optimal execution of the operation. During the procedure, the equivalent of a "black box" will continuously monitor performance and provide feedback information and suggestions (a "virtual mentor"), as well as record the performance of the surgeon's motions and the coordination of the operative team; all of these data will become automatically available as a quantitative record of the surgery to provide continuous documentation for quality improvement, patient safety, and MOC.

SUMMARY

New methods of surgical education, skills training, and assessment, as well as simulation, are just beginning to be incorporated into the fabric of surgery. This innovation represents a true revolution in education, and will set the framework for the next century of surgical education. It is critical that an enormous effort be expended to ensure that a uniformity of approach and quality of training emerges, preventing the fragmented process of education that exists. If we do not achieve such interaction, it will be another century before such an opportunity occurs.

These changes must be implemented across all disciplines and incorporated in laboratory training, in situ training, and daily clinical practice to a point at which simulation becomes automatically embedded in the very culture of surgery. The reward for such an extraordinary effort will be unprecedented levels of quality of care and patient safety.

REFERENCES

1. Seymour NE, Gallagher AG, Roman SA, et al. Virtual reality training improves operating room performance: results of a randomized, double-blinded study. Ann Surg 2002;236:458–64.
2. Flexner A. Medical education in the United States and Canada: a report to the Carnegie Foundation for the Advancement of Teaching (1910). Original document. Available at: http://www.carnegiefoundation.org/files/elibrary/flexner_report.pdf. Accessed November 19, 2009.
3. Resnick R, Regehr G, MacRae H, et al. Testing technical skill via an innovative bench station examination. Am J Surg 1997;173:226–30.

4. Derossis AM, Fried GM, Abrahamowicz M, et al. Development of a model of evaluation and training of laparoscopic skills. Am J Surg 1998;175:482–7.
5. Satava RM. Virtual reality surgical simulator: the first steps. Surg Endosc 1993;7: 203–5.
6. American Council on Graduate Medical Education (ACGME). Program Requirements for Graduate Medical Education in Surgery: Common Program Requirement, Effective: January 1, 2008, Section II D (2). p. 10. Available at: http://www.acgme.org/acWebsite/downloads/RRC_progReq/440_general_surgery_01012008_u08102008.pdf; 2009. Accessed November 19, 2009.
7. American Board of Surgery (ABS). Booklet of information for certifying exam (2009). p. 14. Available at: http://home.absurgery.org/xfer/BookletofInfo-Surgery.pdf. Accessed November 19, 2009.
8. American Board of Pediatrics Maintenance of Certification. Available at: https://www.abp.org/ABPWebStatic/#murl%3D%2FABPWebStatic%2Fmoc.html%26surl%3Dhttps%3A%2F%2Fwww.abp.org%2Fabpwebsite%2Fmoc%2Fphysicianrequirements%2Fquickguides%2Fpermanentcertificates.htm. Accessed November 19, 2009.
9. Mutter D, Dallemagne B, Bailey C, et al. 3-D virtual reality and selective vascular control for laparoscopic left hepatic lobectomy. Surg Endosc 2009;23:432–5.
10. Kahol K, Satava RM, Ferrara J, et al. Effect of short-term pretrial practice on surgical proficiency in simulated environments: a randomized trial of the "preoperative warm-up" effect. J Am Coll Surg 2009;208(2):255–68.

Index

Note: Page numbers of article titles are in **boldface** type.

A

Accreditation Council for Graduate Medical Education (ACGME), 491
ACGME. See *Accreditation Council for Graduate Medical Education (ACGME)*.
ACS Education Institute accreditation process, 501
ACS/APDS National Skills Curriculum, interns skills training, 511, 514–515
Animal/cadaver models of simulators, 462
Anxiety, performance, assessment of, in simulation proficiency, 484
Assessment
    cognitive, in FLS program, reliability and validity of, 544
    in skills laboratory and operating room, **519–533**
        components in need of assessment, 520
        environment for, 522–524
        eye tracking in, 529–530
        feasibility in, 522
        formative assessment, 520
        global rating scales in, 526–527
        importance of, 519–520
        motion tracking in, 527–529
        new technologies in, 529–530
        NIRS in, 529
        observational rating scales in, 526
        procedure for, 522–524
        procedure-specific scales in, 527
        quality of, 521–522
        rating scales of nontechnical performance in, 527
        reliability in, 521
        simulation models, 524–526
            cadaveric models, 524–525
            physical models, 524
            synthetic models, 525
            virtual reality models, 525–526
        summative assessment, 520
        surgical innovation in, 530
        tools in, 526–527
        types of, 520
        validity in, 521–522
Automaticity, in simulation proficiency, 482–483

C

Certification, stimulation in, 619–621
Clinical experience, prerequisites for, verification of proficiency, **559–567**

Surg Clin N Am 90 (2010) 635–641
doi:10.1016/S0039-6109(10)00063-0
0039-6109/10/$ – see front matter © 2010 Elsevier Inc. All rights reserved.

surgical.theclinics.com

Moving?

Make sure your subscription moves with you!

To notify us of your new address, find your **Clinics Account Number** (located on your mailing label above your name), and contact customer service at:

Email: journalscustomerservice-usa@elsevier.com

800-654-2452 (subscribers in the U.S. & Canada)
314-447-8871 (subscribers outside of the U.S. & Canada)

Fax number: 314-447-8029

Elsevier Health Sciences Division
Subscription Customer Service
3251 Riverport Lane
Maryland Heights, MO 63043

*To ensure uninterrupted delivery of your subscription, please notify us at least 4 weeks in advance of move.

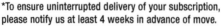

Printed and bound by CPI Group (UK) Ltd, Croydon, CR0 4YY

03/10/2024

01040444-0018